HIV and Depression:
Context and Care

Francisco J González MD

UCSF AIDS Health Project Monograph Series Number Five
Published by the AIDS Health Project, University of California San Francisco
Monograph Series Editors: James W. Dilley, MD and Robert Marks

LIBRARY OF CONGRESS CATALOGING-IN-PUBLICATION DATA

    González, Francisco J. (Francisco José), 1959-

        HIV and depression : context and care / Francisco J. González.

          p. ; cm. -- (UCSF AIDS Health Project monograph series ; no. 5)

        Includes bibliographical references and index.

        ISBN 1-879168-05-7 (pbk.)

          1. HIV-positive persons--Mental health. 2. Depression, Mental--Treatment.

    3. HIV infections--Psychological aspects. I. AIDS Health Project. II. Title. III. Series.

        [DNLM: 1. Depression--etiology. 2. HIV Infections--complications. 3. Anti-depressive Psychotherapy--methods. WC 503.5 G643h 2000]

        RC606.6 .G66 2000

        616.85'27--dc21

                                         00-054506

UCSF AIDS HEALTH PROJECT, Box 0884, San Francisco, CA 94143-0884.

James W. Dilley, MD, Executive Director, Editor. Joanna Rinaldi, Deputy Director. Robert Marks, Manager of Publications, Editor. Saul Rosenfield, Book design, Cover design, Production. Sayre Van Young, Indexing. Kathy Barr, Carrel Crawford, Shauna O'Donnell, Proofreading. Carrel Crawford, Cassia Stepak, Administrative support and distribution. Alex Chase, Beth Fine, Sahar Khoury, Carla Stelling, Cassia Stepak, Research and production support.

The AIDS Health Project is an affiliated unit of the Langley Porter Psychiatric Institute, School of Medicine, University of California San Francisco.

DONATIONS AND GRANTS. Typefaces donated by Adobe Systems, Mountain View, California. We thank Adobe for its generosity.

Funding for this book granted by the California Department of Mental Health: Gray Davis, Governor; Grantland Johnson, Secretary, Health and Welfare Agency; Stephen W. Mayberg, PHD, Director of Mental Health, California Department of Mental Health.

DISCLAIMER. Names used in case scenarios in this book are fictitious.

Contents

UCSF AIDS Health Project Monographs

THE UCSF AIDS HEALTH PROJECT, affiliated with the Langley Porter Psychiatric Institute of the University of California San Francisco's world-renowned medical school, is a leader in developing clinical services and professional education to meet the mental health needs of people affected by HIV disease. Since 1984, The AIDS Health Project has been nationally recognized for pioneering programs in a variety of areas, including HIV-related counseling and support, antibody testing and counseling, and HIV-related substance abuse services.

The UCSF AIDS Health Project Monograph Series, underwritten by the California Department of Mental Health, offers clear, concise, and practical information on HIV-related topics of particular concern to mental health providers. The first four books in the series are: *AIDS and the Impact of Cognitive Impairment: A Treatment Guide for Mental Health Providers* ($7.95); *The Alcohol and Drug Wildcard: Substance Use and Psychiatric Problems in People with HIV* ($9.95); *Working with AIDS Bereavement: A Comprehensive Approach for Mental Health Providers* ($10.95); and *HIV Treatment: Mental Health Aspects of Antiviral Therapy* ($10.95).

UCSF AIDS Health Project Publications

THE UCSF AIDS HEALTH PROJECT publishes a range of other publications for mental health and health care providers. The AIDS Health Project published what has become a standard in HIV counseling primers, *Face to Face: A Guide to AIDS Counseling* ($16.95). In late 1998, AHP joined with Jossey-Bass Publishers, Inc. to publish a successor to this volume: *The UCSF AIDS Health Project Guide to Counseling: Perspectives on Psychotherapy, Prevention, and Therapeutic Practice* ($27.95; direct price).

In addition, AHP has published other books for mental health providers, including: *Risk and Recovery: AIDS, HIV, and Alcohol* ($16.95) and *AIDS Law for Mental Health Professionals: A Guide to Judicious Practice* ($19.95).

Finally, AHP publishes several newsletters, including *FOCUS: A Guide to AIDS Research and Counseling*, one of the longest-running HIV-related newsletters in the country. *FOCUS*, which has an international reputation, reviews the counseling aspects of HIV disease and is an indispensible reference for counselors, health care providers, and scholars ($36.00 for an individual subscription; $90.00 for an institutional subscription; international rates available). AHP also publishes *HIV Counselor PERSPECTIVES*, a newsletter for antibody test counselors ($24.00 for an individual subscription; $60.00 for an institutional subscription; international rates available).

For more information or to order AHP publications, please write UCSF AIDS Health Project, Box 0884, San Francisco, CA 94143-0884; call 415-502-4930; fax 415-476-7996; or visit our web site: www.ucsf-ahp.org.

About the Author

FRANCISCO J. GONZÁLEZ, MD is Assistant Clinical Professor of Psychiatry at the University of California San Francisco and Medical Director at Instituto Familiar de la Raza, a Latino community service organization. He has worked with HIV since the early 1980s and has written and presented on a variety of issues at the intersections of Latino culture, homosexuality, and HIV.

Acknowledgments

Putting a monograph like this together requires the efforts of many people. The author and the editors extend their appreciation to UCSF AIDS Health Project staff and volunteers who contributed to the process. (See the copyright page for a list of these individuals.) In addition, the authors wish to especially acknowledge the following people.

Writing is always a collaborative process. In this project, several people deserve mention. Beth Fine, an intern at the UCSF AIDS Health Project (AHP), helped with research assistance. George Harrison, MD at AHP and Nan O'Connor, LCSW at the Center for Special Problems reviewed the manuscript and provided useful comments that steered it in the right direction. Rob Marks and Jim Dilley, as editors, were patient and consistently helpful, pruning and watering as needed. The greatest debt I owe is to the many clients with HIV with whom I've had the privilege to work. I deeply respect their struggle and admire their perseverance, fortitude, and resilience. They are my foremost teachers.

Introduction

Depression has been associated with human immunodeficiency virus (HIV) infection from the very beginning of the epidemic. To some, depression must still seem the only possible response to an illness that can devastate psychological and social – as well as physical – integrity. Who would not be depressed by the loss of bodily control and by being marked by a disease of almost mythic proportions? Yet the responses of individuals to the enormous challenges of living with HIV are disparate: while some people collapse in resignation and despair or become eerily indifferent, others seem to come alive, manifesting an inner strength and resolve. Nor are these states fixed: HIV infection initiates a long and complicated emotional process during which there are often moments of despair, of denial, but also of strength, even heroism. This unfolding process necessarily includes moments of sadness and personal loss. But when does such a depressive response become significant enough to warrant mental health intervention?

One cannot work with people with HIV and be insensitive to the inevitability of profound loss. But this sensitivity cannot blind providers to the possibility of intervention. This monograph provides practical guidelines to the process of diagnosing and treating depression in people with HIV, without diminishing the complexity of these challenges.

The Historical Context of HIV

To understand depression in the context of HIV, it is useful to understand HIV in the context of its history. In the early 1980s, the first years of the epidemic in the United States, science could offer very little in the way of treatment or even social support. At the outset, the disease did not have a name, its agent and the mode of transmission were unknown, and it was invariably fatal. In urban epicenters, gay and bisexual men fell seriously ill, were diagnosed, and died, often within a year after presenting for medical care. Some were diagnosed with AIDS only after watching their closest friends sicken and die. Many in the so-called high-risk groups (primarily gay and bisexual men and injection drug users) felt a sense of inevitability, guilt, fear, and hopelessness, and ultimately a state of sustained bereavement fed by the repeated trauma of loss. Such accumulated loss could easily result in depression, demoralization, and numbness. It was not uncommon to find "burn out" among informal and professional caregivers, as wave upon wave of casualties exhausted psychological reserves. Hopelessness, exacerbated by a lack of information, characterized that confusing and anxiety-ridden time.

The U.S. Food and Drug Administration (FDA) approved the HIV antibody test in 1985, it was not until the late 1980s that it approved zidovudine (ZDV; AZT), the first HIV antiviral treatment. Up to that point, treatment for opportunistic conditions offered little more than a temporary postponement of illness. By 1990, early hopes about the promise of ZDV met with disappointment.

By the mid-1980s, reports began to indicate elevated levels of psychopathology, particularly clinical depression, among people with HIV disease.[1] Suicide rates among people with AIDS were alarmingly high: in one New York City study, 66 times higher than the general population;[2] in a California study, 21 times higher.[3] These early reports may have established an expectation among caregivers that depression was correlated with HIV disease, but closer examination shows that these early studies were often conducted on individuals with advanced illness and at a time when there was little hope. These historical artifacts may continue to color perceptions about the relationship between HIV and depression. While studies have become more sophisticated, the published data on the prevalence of clinical depression and the nature of its relationship to HIV is inconclusive and widely divergent: depression prevalence rates range from 0 percent to 80 percent in HIV-positive populations.[4]

Fortunately, the social and clinical background of the HIV epidemic has changed dramatically since the 1980s. Providers now diagnose HIV infection much closer to the time of seroconversion rather than late in the course of HIV disease, allowing both clients and clinicians to adjust to the illness over time and plan for the eventualities of disease progression. Researchers have slowly developed new and improved treatment options, resulting in greater control both of opportunistic conditions and HIV infection itself. With the advent of multidrug antiviral treatment in the mid-1990s, the psychological landscape of the epidemic changed radically: these new regimens introduced the possibility of managing illness and sustaining quality of life, rather than simply surviving HIV disease. Moribund fatalism has been transformed into nervous hope. In fact, when triple combination treatments were first introduced, some rashly declared the end of the epidemic, a prediction that has lamentably not come to pass. But advances in the late 1990s did end the epidemic as it had been known to that point: the future *has* brightened, although it remains fraught with anxiety and new burdens.

Over the past two decades, HIV-related services have also become more sophisticated and more readily available. AIDS service organizations have developed specialized programs based on the specific needs of the subpopulations most affected by the epidemic: self-identified gay and bisexual men; men who engage in homosexual activity but do not identify as gay; women; transgendered people; people of color; sex workers; injection drug users; and homeless people. (Of course, these subpopulations overlap within themselves.) In a truly unprecedented project of coordination, medical services have been more closely linked with social outreach and mental health programs. Activists who challenged the medical and pharmacological establishments in the 1980s forced dramatic changes in the structure and delivery of services, the development of medication and access to

3

clinical trials, and the setting of state and national policy. If the early 1980s were a time of shock and despair, the late 1980s and early 1990s were a time of response and action, arguably leading to improved mental health conditions. While the statistics are not beyond methodological reproach, by 1992 a national assessment of people with AIDS reported a significant decline in the rate of suicide among men from 10.5 times higher than men in the general population in 1987 to 6.0 times higher in 1989.[5]

Making the Darkness Visible

Suicide rates are at best the grossest markers of depression. While these rates have declined, depression nonetheless remains a common problem in HIV-related practice, probably ranging between 15 percent and 20 percent among people with HIV.[6,7] Even when it is not life-threatening, severe depression causes a significant loss of function and a marked diminishment in quality of life. Close relationships become extremely difficult, straining social networks. Productive work is significantly impaired or made impossible by the mind's sluggishness and its reluctance to focus or attend. Individuals suffering from depression often describe it as a bleak prison, a deadening and painful heaviness that entraps by infiltrating every moment and aspect of their lives. A person's very relationship to the sense of self becomes distorted, so that rather than feeling compassion or pity for one's predicament, a person suffering from clinical depression often feels a pervasive attitude of self-castigation and disgust. To make matters worse, the usual avenues an individual might use to help him or herself feel better – contact with others, pleasurable distractions, nurturing indulgence – become closed off by isolation, a lack of motivation, and an absence of pleasure. The experience of depression is indeed a deeply painful one, a "darkness visible," as writer William Styron has called it.[8]

Beyond these damaging psychological effects, depression can also influence physical well-being. Whether there is a direct link between HIV disease progression and clinical levels of depression remains unclear. For example, while controlling for immune status and markers of HIV disease progression, one study found that depression, but not other accompanying health conditions, led to a higher risk of progression to an AIDS diagnosis.[9] The reasons why depression might contribute to progression are many and unproven.

It is conceivable, however, that depressed individuals might be less likely to seek medical attention or to follow self-care recommendations. Self-care is a critical component of maintaining health in HIV disease, and depression typically erodes the nurturing relationship to oneself. A Pittsburgh Veterans Administration Medical Center study significantly correlated high rates of adherence to HIV medication regimens (defined as taking 80 percent or more of prescribed medications) with lower levels of depression, better adaptive coping, and diminished psychological disturbance.[10] In a general medical study (not specific to HIV), researchers found that depressed patients were three times as likely as non-depressed patients to be nonadherent to medical treatment recommendations.[11]

Yet, despite the high rates of depression and its clinical significance, many providers and clients fail to recognize depression when it occurs. In a survey of 475 HIV-infected men without AIDS, for example, researchers found that clinical depression was seriously undertreated: of the 176 men (37 percent of the entire sample) who demonstrated significant symptoms of depression, only 40 percent had seen a mental health clinician in the previous year, and only about 6 percent were taking antidepressant medications.[12] Why, in an age when depression is the subject of talk shows and national bestsellers, should this be the case?

The answer may have to do with the complex and confusing relationship between depression and HIV disease, in part a result of the epidemic's history of uncertainty and despair and the distorting shadow it casts on current clinical situations. Consider the following questions. Isn't it normal for someone who has a life-threatening illness to feel depressed? Rather than calling attention to depressive feelings, isn't it better to put them aside and get on with living? Aren't complaints of fatigue and decreased motivation more properly attributable to the malaise and other physical symptoms of HIV disease rather than to a "mental condition"?

There are also other, perhaps more academic or scientific, questions that confuse this issue. Does HIV progression predispose an individual to depressive disorders? Conversely, does depression promote immune system malfunction and illness progression? What is the relationship between the stress and trauma of HIV-related events such as initial diagnosis or the development of symptoms and other life traumas? Does depression significantly contribute to high-risk sexual activity? Do different groups at risk for HIV have different rates or kinds of depression?

Finally, for medical providers caring for HIV-positive patients, there are a host of other concerns. How do I recognize clinical depression and differentiate it from other symptoms of HIV disease? What can I do to help an individual who is depressed? What are the best ways to treat depression in HIV-positive clients? When should I refer a client to a mental health provider for treatment of depression?

Monograph Overview: Clarifying Confusion

The purpose of this monograph is to clarify the confusion that often surrounds the assessment and treatment of depressive symptoms in the context of HIV disease – without becoming formulaic or oversimplistic. Specifically, the monograph seeks to focus on depression within a human context, a context that does not sacrifice social and cultural understanding for reductionist medicalization. To accomplish this, the monograph defines the assessment and treatment of depression in terms of the contexts in which they occur: the context of normal sadness versus clinical depression; the context of cultural factors that play out in the therapeutic relationship; and the context of the care venues in which depression may arise.

Depression is a protean, multifaceted phenomenon resulting from complex and often interacting causes. Indeed, the generic rubric of "depression" actually includes several different formal psychiatric diagnoses as well as a range of normal responses. Because of this complexity, this monograph strives to focus on clinical realities, recognizing that individual clients present with complaints, not with neat diagnostic categories. These complaints are often characterized by a confusing amalgam of fuzzy symptoms and unrelated signs. The monograph conceptualizes depression as a spectrum with a broad range, its endpoints located in everyday transient sadness at one end and suicidal crisis at the other. Providers must locate a client's condition along this spectrum by analyzing clinical phenomena – the client's symptoms and his or her interactions with the clinical context – a process that allows a more complete understanding of depression than one that routinely medicalizes depressive symptoms. There are times when depressive feelings are both natural and necessary and need to be given room to resolve themselves, and other times when they are malignant and eroding, and should be aggressively rooted out.

Depression manifests in various ways ranging from the client's subjective narrative of "what's wrong" to more objective physical dysfunctions such as changes in appetite or in the quickness of routine movements. In whatever way a client expresses depressive symptoms, however, it is always in the context of a relationship with a provider. Both individuals in this pairing – the client and the provider – are embedded in an intersection of rich cultural matrices: the culture of an institution or clinic or discipline; an ethnic, religious, racial, or immigrant culture; a culture of sexuality and gender; or a culture of drugs or the street. A principle thesis of the monograph is that cultural factors play an essential role in the particular manifestations of depression and so should constitute a determining force for providers in assessment and treatment planning.

Finally, psychiatric disorders and psychological symptoms do not occur in a vacuum, any more so than do viral load levels or CD4+ cell counts. If anything, it has long been apparent that issues as disparate as housing, social support, financial resources, and psychological resiliency are as critical to the successful outcome of a medical treatment plan as are state-of-the-art antiviral treatments and good nutrition. These days, HIV disease management is often carried out by a team of providers who attend to these various needs. Recognition and treatment of clinical depression constitutes a critical intervention in this spectrum of care. As such, this monograph is aimed at a wide variety of HIV providers, including mental health practitioners, HIV primary care clinicians, and social service providers.

The monograph designates specific psychiatric diagnoses of depression following standard nomenclature as defined by the *Diagnostic and Statistical Manual of Mental Disorders, Fourth Edition* (DSM-IV), for example, major depressive disorder, dysthymia, and so forth.[13] By grouping detailed symptom clusters, DSM-IV diagnoses offer clinicians efficient ways to think and communicate about complicated information. These diagnoses are indispensable tools for assessment, treatment, and research. When referring to depressive symptoms that are severe enough to warrant diagnosis along the lines of DSM-IV criteria, the monograph uses the generic term "clinical depression." As outlined above, not all depressive symptomatology attains the level of clinical depression.

The monograph is divided into four chapters. Chapter One presents the concept of depression as a spectrum of symptoms that range from normal to those constituting a clinical disorder. This chapter reinforces the biopsychosocial model of understanding psychiatric disturbance and applies it in the context of HIV. It also examines general methodological difficulties involved in determining the prevalence of HIV-related clinical depression. Chapter Two outlines important variables in the assessment of depression, including sociocultural, psychological, and medical confounds that complicate an understanding of HIV-related depression. It returns to the prevalence literature on clinical depression to examine studies pertaining to various subpopulations affected by the epidemic – gay men, injection drug users, people of color, and women. This chapter emphasizes the critical importance of understanding the context of depressive phenomena. Chapter Three defines an approach for the assessment of depression, including a review of the DSM criteria for a major depressive episode and the differential diagnosis of clinical depressions. Chapter Four presents treatment interventions and strategies, including the use of antidepressant medications and a review of important psychotherapeutic approaches. Each chapter draws from the scientific literature as appropriate and provides illustrative clinical case material and vignettes.

Over time, the HIV epidemic has unquestionably inflicted a trauma concentrated in particular communities. It is natural and healthy to express distress in the face of such devastation, but providers and their clients are by no means helpless in the face of depression. This monograph seeks to provide some direction for those struggling against the tide of loss imposed by HIV.

1
Defining Depression

DEPRESSION is an unwieldy and imprecise concept that can encompass a number of specific psychiatric diagnoses – or none at all. The term can be used casually to describe an innocuous variation in daily mood, and it can suggest the sadness that accompanies normal grief over loss. As such, depression can be normal, even necessary. Not infrequently clients use the term to mean a number of mental states, ranging from a difficulty in initiating and executing plans to sustained emotional conditions of nervousness, sadness, frustration, or anger. As a diagnosable psychiatric entity, depression can be circumstantial, a response to specific traumatic events, or it can arise without clear precipitating antecedents. It can manifest as a secondary symptom of another disorder, such as a variety of medical illnesses, like hypothyroidism, or it can represent its own significant primary psychiatric disorder. When a client complains of "depression," the clinician may find him or herself facing a combination of many possible conditions, states, and emotional problems.

For the clinician, the practical questions are: when do I intervene and how do I intervene? To make these determinations, it is
important first to find a way of describing and defining a client's
"depression," to conceptualize it along the continuum of distress and
function. Clinicians are better prepared to do this if they have some
background on the ways of defining depression in general, its etiology, and how it is discussed within the HIV literature.

A Grouping of Symptoms

What do we really mean when we employ this commonplace
term with so many possible designations? This monograph uses the
general term "depression" to designate a symptom or group of
symptoms, rather than a specific diagnosis. This approach is consistent with clinical realities: clients often present with vague complaints of "being down" or "not feeling right." It falls to the provider
to elicit a history of symptoms, evaluate confounding variables such
as substance use or fatigue due to illness, analyze the data at hand,
and form preliminary diagnoses and treatment plans. This clinical
enterprise can be daunting in the context of HIV disease. For example, the clinician may have to consider the alienating impact on a
client of a new self-concept such as "AIDS patient" and differentiate
the isolation resulting from that effect from the apathy that can
accompany HIV-associated dementia. He or she may have to sort out
the depressive effects of a client's occasional amphetamine use from
the protracted bereavement following the death of the client's partner. In short, clinicians need to understand how to work with both
the social and the biological, and how these forces interact and
express themselves in the context of the client's psychological reality.

For the purposes of this monograph, and consonant with client-
centered approaches, a depressive symptom is determined by the
client's subjective experience of having an emotional problem: the
client reports a sense that something is wrong, that there is a malfunction in daily living. Seen in this light, a depressive symptom describes a
relative change for the client, not an absolute level of functioning. An
individual may successfully work forty hours a week and have many
supportive relationships, but he or she may still experience symptomatic depression if it diminishes efficiency at work or deteriorates the
quality of relationships. The classic depressive symptoms are sadness
or a lack of pleasure, decreased motivation (also called inanition), and

an apathetic despair characterized by hopelessness and helplessness. Clients may report uncontrollable crying spells or a sense of feeling "stuck" in their psychological lives, but they can also present with more subtle complaints such as a vague disconnectedness from significant others, weight loss, or forgetfulness and difficulty concentrating.

Sometimes depressive symptoms can be latent, effectively hidden from view. To express depressive feeling is to be vulnerable, and for some this state of vulnerability and relative dependence feels dangerous and troubling. Such clients struggle against the undertow of negative emotions, turning to reckless behavior, alcohol and drug use, promiscuity, or angry encounters as a way to distance themselves from depressive feelings or to hide these feelings from others. What shows on the surface can be diametrically opposed to the expected reactions of sadness or withdrawal. These latent depressive symptoms often emerge only over time, as the client comes to trust the provider more deeply and can risk greater vulnerability, or as the defensive strategies fail and the depressive symptoms burst into the open.

Probably almost all individuals with HIV, at one time or another, experience depressive symptoms. These are natural responses to loss, and HIV disease (whether asymptomatic or severe) opens the door to a variety of losses. Illness brings the obvious loss of function, well-being, and comfort, but HIV can also mean the loss of identity or social standing. In response, symptoms of distress naturally include intense sadness, anger, anxiety, and frustration. In distress, the individual is usually hurting but usually not hurting him or herself: self-care generally remains intact, and there is a sense of what to do next, of how to continue. These depressive symptoms are difficult, but manageable. When symptoms of distress reach the threshold of significantly impairing psychological and social function, an individual enters the world of clinical depression. Symptoms of a clinical depression are more severe and can include weight loss, insomnia, self-deprecation, and suicidal ideation.

The markers used to divide distress from clinical depression are fluid, contextual, and ultimately arbitrary. Crying intensely on learning one has seroconverted might be a marker of distress, but at what point does it become a sign of clinical depression: when it happens everyday, when it does not remit after a few days, when it does not remit after two weeks? If a client is suffering from severe peripheral neuropathy (pain in the extremities) it is predictable that he or she will complain and express sadness or frustration. At what point does this complaint indicate that the client is emotionally overtaxed and signaling for help? These concerns have generated a substantial body of academic literature; they are at the heart of what has made understanding depression in the context of HIV confusing.

The Etiology of Depression

Over the years, a number of theories have sought to establish conclusive causes of depression, but none of these has held up under close scientific scrutiny. Today most researchers would probably agree that depression is caused by an interaction of various factors that occur at both biological and psychosocial levels.[14]

One of the earliest theorists of depression was Sigmund Freud. He proposed that depression represented rage turned against the self when an individual experienced the loss of someone dear. Rather than entering mourning – and grieving and relinquishing what was lost – the individual became "melancholic," filled with guilt and self-reproach. In this model of depression, symptoms achieve a disruptive clinical level when the mourning process goes awry and the individual cannot tolerate the experience of grief. This perspective still has utility as a way of understanding cases of complicated bereavement (see Chapter Four). Other psychoanalytic figures further elaborated psychological theories of depression to include the failure to establish loving internal representations towards the self based on a lack of empathic understanding from significant others.

Behavioral scientists have added the concept of learned helplessness, postulating that depression is the manifestation of the sense that a person has no control over a distressing circumstance. In the classic, and somewhat brutal, experiment of learned helplessness, researchers gave animals electric shocks. Struggling initially, the animals ultimately gave in and made no further attempts to escape. In what could be considered an extension of this work, cognitive theorists consider that faulty cognitions – negatively-hued misinterpretations and distortions of the self and the world – result in depressive feelings.

With the advent of medications to effectively treat clinical depression, researchers ushered in a host of biological theories of depression. The most salient of these theories have implicated the "biogenic amines," substances that act as neurotransmitters or chemical messengers between brain cells. The most important of these biogenic amines are norepinephrine and serotonin. Norepinephrine is the neurotransmitter most affected by tricyclic antidepressants such as nortriptyline (Pamelor); serotonin is the neurotransmitter most affected by selective serotonin reuptake inhibitors such as fluoxetine (Prozac). There are complicated interactions among the various amines and other biological factors, including the inheritance of a predisposition to depression.

Finally, theorists suggest that social or environmental factors have a role in causing depression. Studies have found that stressful life events precede first episodes of mood disorders more frequently than subsequent episodes. One explanation is that the initial episode of clinical depression, caused by the stressful event, alters the brain's chemistry, which facilitates later depressive episodes.

One way of viewing this variety of theories is to see them as complementary rather than contradictory. Biological tendencies toward depression are almost certainly inherited, and they are probably mediated through deficiencies in the biogenic amine and other neurotransmitter systems. But this inherited tendency may then be further molded, blunted, or exacerbated, through the early life experiences that help shape personality. A good and loving childhood may increase a sense of self-worth and bolster resiliency, just as traumatic experiences and inconsistent or grossly negligent parenting almost certainly ends in a damaged sense of self. When later stressful life events or traumas affect a person, the infinitely complicated balance of inherited biological predispositions and developed personality may either be strong enough to deal with the new trauma in a way that avoids depression or may collapse under the weight of this trauma and result in clinical symptoms.

Factors Causing HIV-Related Depression

The causes and manifestations of depression in people with HIV are likewise based on the interaction of biological, psychological, and social factors. HIV infection initiates a host of biological responses in the body, and these changes can lead to HIV-related symptoms that can mimic primary depressive syndromes. This process occurs in two ways: as a direct consequence of the viral infection and as a result of secondary – or opportunistic – infections or neoplasms. The primary viral illness associated with HIV infection, for example, can produce fatigue, lethargy, and malaise; as it directly infects the central nervous system (CNS) tissues, HIV causes neuropathies and, in some, HIV-associated dementia. Dementia, characterized by apathy and motor as well as cognitive slowing, can easily imitate depressive syndromes. Other opportunistic diseases that affect the central nervous system – like toxoplasmosis or lymphomas, or even more general opportunistic infections, like *Pneumocystis carinii* pneumonia – can produce significant psychoneurological symptoms that, particularly early in the disease course, may be mistaken for depression. Clients may also suffer from anemia or wasting syndromes that exacerbate fatigue. As if this were not confusing enough, clients with HIV often take complicated medication regimens that can result in a myriad of side effects. All of these biological processes may appear to both client and clinician as manifestations of clinical depression, or conversely, symptoms of a significant clinical depression may be "explained away" as merely logical consequences of being sick.

But it is the psychological plane that is of most concern for the mental health practitioner, and the one through which other information is often mediated. When confronted by the biological or emotional vicissitudes of their bodies, clients tell providers their stories about what they think and feel is going on inside. These narratives are colored by an individual's character or personality, and each client creates a specific psychological language for relating his or her pain to the provider. Different personality types will manage traumatic material in different ways. One individual may become withdrawn and uncommunicative; another may become emotionally voluble, angry, and attacking; others may feel suspicious and wary or, conversely, dependent and needy. Every client comes to HIV disease with a specific and personal history. How the current depressive episode fits into this life story, how the individual relates it to HIV, and what depression and HIV – even health and illness – mean to him or her: these questions constitute an essential part of understanding the client as a whole.

Finally, the individual is embedded in a social and cultural matrix of relationships with partners and family, friends, and the larger community. For some, these relationships reflect supportive ties, for others, they act as constraints. In some cases, these bonds are notably absent. At this social level, too, salient factors shape the manifestation of depression. In the United States, HIV disease came to prominence with an association to gay men and slightly later to injection drug users, both marginalized and stigmatized groups. Too many in these groups are literally the last survivors of their circle of friends after the devastation of the 1980s. More recently, the epidemic has advanced along sociodemographically distinguishable lines into communities of color, and particularly among women of color. These communities are often already disadvantaged, armed with relatively few resources and impeded in their access to health care. HIV remains the illness that dares not speak its name, and the fear of rejection imposes an isolating silence. Social bonds form part of the fabric against which depression unfolds, and the stigmatizing and socially-disruptive nature of HIV can thin that fabric, leaving individuals more exposed and vulnerable.

When it becomes severe enough to significantly disrupt normal function, depression constitutes an illness. At that point, it almost always cuts across biological, psychological, and social planes. There are three such depressive illnesses designated in the DSM-IV: "major depressive disorder," "dysthymia," and "depressive disorder not otherwise specified." At the heart of a diagnosis of major depression is the prototypical major depressive episode. A diagnosis of major depression includes the presence of a major depressive episode and excludes bipolar disorder (manic-depression) and psychotic disorders. Dysthymia is a milder form of major depression, but typically more chronic (lasting at least two years). The "not otherwise specified" (NOS) diagnosis includes atypical depressions. (See Chapter Three for diagnostic criteria for these depressive conditions and their differential diagnosis.)

But these are not the only formal diagnoses that include primarily depressive symptoms, and certainly not the only ones encountered by HIV providers. In addition to the effects of illness already noted above, alcohol, street drugs, and sedative/hypnotic medications can all cause depressive disorders. Psychologically significant or frankly traumatic events can also catalyze the development of adjustment disorders with depressive symptoms. Adjustment disorders are common in HIV-related practice, and while usually less severe and of shorter duration than major depressive episodes, they nonetheless cause significant impairment in functioning. Finally, certain personality disorders, marked by interpersonal strife and isolation, may result in depressive syndromes.

Determining the Prevalence of Depression

Many studies have been conducted to determine the prevalence – the rate of depression at any given time – among people with HIV. These studies have compared HIV-positive asymptomatic individuals with those with full-blown AIDS, often along the lines of ethnicity, gender, race, sexuality, or method of transmission. For at least the last fifteen years, researchers have been struggling with the question of whether HIV disease effectively predisposes individuals to clinical depression, and the controversy is still not settled. Why has it been so difficult to come up with a definitive answer? A review of the literature suggests four factors that may compromise the prevalence data.

First, depression prevalence studies can examine only a limited sample of any given population, and it is difficult to generalize from these samples to larger populations. Among the traditional "at-risk" groups, the most frequently studied have been White gay and bisexual men, a group with significant psychosocial differences from injection drug users, women, other racial or ethnic groups, and the homeless and chronically mentally ill populations. Differences in gender, ethnicity, economic status, and coexisting medical or psychiatric illness can significantly affect prevalence rates. Rates of HIV-related depression among homeless injection drug users and middle class White gay men, for example, might be predicted to vary considerably. Such differences in prevalence might be intrinsic to the populations, or they could be an artifact of methodological problems in recruiting subjects, or they could be due to variations in each population's access to health care. Nor are the subgroups sampled themselves homogeneous. Enormous variety exists within a given group of women, gay men, or African Americans. Moreover, group designations are not exclusive, but rather frequently overlap, as in Latino bisexual men or homeless women of color who use injection drugs. Finally, most studies use "convenience sampling," recruiting subjects from community centers, through newspaper ads, or by word of mouth. Subjects in early studies were often recruited from clinics, and clinic patients may differ in rates of depression from individuals not attending clinics. In short, sampling methods cannot ensure that a cohort represents the general population of HIV-infected people.

Second, prevalence studies employ a variety of standardized measurement tools to assess depression. Differences in these tools can result in substantial discrepancies in prevalence rates. While some studies rely on self-report by the study subject – who fills out a standardized form such as the Beck Depression Inventory (BDI) or the Centers for Epidemiological Studies Depression Scale (CES-D) – other studies use interviewer-administered tools. Symptomatic individuals might endorse symptoms of depression on self-report measures that may more appropriately be ascribed to medical illness by a trained interviewer asking clarifying questions. In fact, many self-report rating scales used in research on depression and HIV (for example, the BDI and the Minnesota Multiphasic Personality Inventory (MMPI)) contain items assessing vegetative or somatic symptoms of depression that may artificially elevate depression scores by inappropriately interpreting medical symptoms as depressive ones. A number of studies have demonstrated the confounding overlap between somatic symptoms of HIV and depression in these self-report tools.[15-19]

Third, most studies of the prevalence of depression in people with HIV have been cross-sectional, that is, they compare two groups of individuals (seropositive subjects and seronegative controls) at a particular point in time. Such studies cannot answer questions of causation, since there is no way to determine if depression preceded or followed the effects of HIV disease. These studies merely demonstrate an association between HIV and depression. HIV disease may have led to depression, or depression may have put an individual at greater risk of contracting HIV (for example, by leading to unsafe sex), or depression may be associated with a third variable such as having male homosexual sex, which itself is statistically associated with HIV status.

Finally, the question of causality is complicated by confusion in the definition of depression from study to study. As previously noted, depression means many things to many people, including scientific investigators. In their editorial, "Depressive Syndromes and Causal Associations," HIV researchers Constantine Lyketsos and Glenn Treisman argue that prevalence rates of depression in the context of HIV disease fluctuate so widely because researchers differ in their conceptions of depression – defining it variously as an affect, a symptom, or a full clinical syndrome – and in their causal attribution of such "depression" to the general medical condition of HIV.[20] Whether a common scientific language will eventually evolve remains to be seen; but whatever happens, studies to date remain inconsistent in their terminology. Because of these complex methodological problems, it is difficult to interpret prevalence studies on HIV-related depression, and often impossible to compare one study to another.

General Studies on Depression Prevalence

Two relatively recent, general studies of the prevalence of depression do offer a useful overview. The World Health Organization (WHO) undertook a survey of five cities – Bangkok, Kinshasa, Munich, Nairobi, and São Paulo – as representative of the areas most affected by the epidemic.[21] Published in 1996, the study provides an overall view of the relation between depression and HIV in a well-controlled, methodologically rigorous design. Researchers used a series of assessment tools, including neuropsychological batteries and a structured, psychiatric interview. The study did not differentiate participants in terms of risk group attribution, but rather recruited subjects consecutively from outpatient clinics. The result is that some risk groups are prominent at some sites but not at others: for example, the Bangkok sample is overwhelmingly composed of injection drug users, while the Munich sample is quite mixed, including gay and bisexual men, injection drug users, and blood transfusion recipients.

The WHO study found that rates of major depression for symptomatic HIV-positive individuals ranged from 4 percent in Munich to 18 percent in Bangkok. For those with asymptomatic HIV, the rates were lower, ranging from 0 percent in Kinshasa to 11 percent in São Paulo. Although not statistically significant, there was a trend for HIV-positive individuals to have higher rates of major depression than HIV-negative individuals. In its evaluation of depressive symptoms, in contrast to the full diagnosis of major depression, however, the study found a statistically significant difference between individuals with symptomatic disease and seronegative individuals. The author of the study concludes:

> The results of the WHO Neuropsychiatric AIDS Study suggest that the symptomatic stages of HIV infection are associated with an increased prevalence of depressive symptoms, and, at least in some contexts in which the spreading of the infection is more recent and the social rejection of HIV-seropositive subjects is harsher, may also be associated with an increased prevalence of a syndromal diagnosis of depression.[21]

This conclusion brings together the relationship between symptoms and sociocultural factors, and demonstrates how stressors from an illness could result in a full-fledged psychiatric disorder (with a corresponding impairment in function) if there is not adequate social support. In fact, the author suggests that the reason U.S.-based studies of gay and bisexual men have not found significant differences in depression rates between HIV-positive and HIV-negative subjects is that the convenience sampling often used in these studies selects those men who are most connected to the gay community and, therefore, most likely to have the social support that might protect against depression.

A second general study, published in 1997, compared cohorts of HIV-positive and HIV-negative men in the United States over a period of one year.[22] Researchers attempted the ambitious task of recruiting all the seropositive people in a metropolitan area who were seen in primary care settings. They identified the principal HIV physicians in the area and asked these physicians to approach each of their HIV-positive patients. Since the study enrolled relatively few women, researchers conducted analyses only on men. They measured depression at baseline and subsequently at six- and twelve-month intervals.

The study found no statistically significant difference in lifetime rates of major depression or dysthymia for the two groups: rates of major depression were 48 percent for HIV-positive men and 37 percent for HIV-negative men; rates of dysthymia were 9 percent and 4 percent, respectively. After twelve months, however, rates of major depression for the HIV-positive group differed significantly from those of the seronegative control group: 37 percent for HIV-positive men and 15 percent for HIV-negative men. Both lifetime and current rates of major depression were higher for all subjects than for the general population. (In addition, seropositive men differed significantly from seronegative men for two other psychiatric diagnoses: adjustment disorder with anxiety and substance abuse or dependence.) The authors also analyzed risk factors for the development of psychiatric disorders. Results demonstrated that younger age, a history of major depression, and low levels of support from household members all correlated with a diagnosis of major depression. These effects were independent of other variables such as demographics. Additionally, seropositive men who had known about their HIV infection for less time and those who were recently diagnosed with AIDS were at increased risk of depression, confirming the common sense expectation that such stressors can make clients especially vulnerable to depressive illness.

Both the WHO and U.S. study employ representative, rather than convenience, sampling, which strengthens their methodology and increases their generalizability. While they provide no definitive statement as to the prevalence of depressive disorders among people with HIV disease, they do indicate that under carefully controlled conditions, it can be shown that an AIDS diagnosis, and perhaps symptomatic HIV disease, but not HIV infection alone, may predispose individuals to clinical depression. The controversy surrounding these findings suggests a more important issue for front-line practitioners: depressive symptoms are modulated by a number of complex and interacting variables. The degree of social connectedness and support, a psychiatric history of depression, age and risk-group membership, social and cultural factors: all influence the ability to make clear determinations about the relationship of HIV and depression. For clinicians, who encounter individuals rather than abstractions, this complexity underscores the importance of conducting careful assessments.

Juan: Significant Loss of Function

A clinical vignette, based on an actual case history, illustrates some of the complexities outlined above. The case of "Juan" – a 52-year-old, bilingual, single, seropositive gay man from Central America – provides an overview of the entire spectrum of treatment, from presentation and assessment through formulation to intervention. Subsequent chapters offer a more detailed look at the various stages of this process.

Juan was referred to mental health services by a social worker at his primary medical clinic after he complained of depression and poor functioning. Juan had lost 15 pounds in two months, experienced many vague aches and pains, and was apathetic. His contact with his primary care provider – a non-Spanish-speaking White physician with a busy practice – was irregular at best, and although it was clear his health was deteriorating, Juan was reluctant to pursue a medical work-up. Previous routine blood tests had revealed a mild anemia, a CD4+ cell count of 75, and a viral load of 350,000. Several attempts to initiate an aggressive HIV antiviral treatment had failed, largely because Juan had trouble adhering to drug regimens. Because of his physical deterioration, he had recently been placed in hospice care.

On his first visit to the medical clinic's psychiatrist, Juan appeared disheveled and moved slowly. He could not sustain eye contact and seemed unconcerned about his well-being. He acknowledged the breakup of a seven-month-long relationship and complained of profound sadness and a sense that he had "wasted his life." While Juan denied overt suicidality, he said that he "didn't care about living any more." He complained of trouble falling asleep and seemed lethargic and fatigued. Preliminary cognitive testing was limited because of Juan's lack of attention, but these tests showed visual-spatial construction deficits and memory and concentration difficulties.

A psychiatric and psychosocial history revealed the following: Juan had come to the United States fleeing poverty at the age of 23. Moving to Los Angeles, where he had distant relatives, he had initially worked odd jobs and experienced great financial hardship. He persisted, ultimately established himself as a tailor, and in his early thirties, he moved to San Francisco, in part to explore a newly-established gay identity. It was there Juan experienced his first bout of depression after the breakup of a long-term romantic relationship. At that time, Juan's chronic feelings of poor self-esteem, guilt, and internalized racism and homophobia escalated. To stave off these feelings, Juan resorted to alcohol, bingeing on weekends to the point of blacking out and sometimes having unprotected anonymous sexual encounters. The depressive symptoms and the alcohol abuse waxed and waned, but Juan did not seek professional help.

It was not until years later, in his mid-forties, that Juan learned he was HIV-positive. In response, Juan became painfully isolated and drank daily. His self-esteem plummeted, and he contemplated hanging himself. When he began to hear voices encouraging the suicide, he called a friend who took him to the local emergency room. This led to an involuntary hospitalization with a diagnosis of major depression with psychotic features. Juan remembers this hospitalization now as "the event that saved my life."

Treating Juan's Depression

Juan's case illustrates the complexity of diagnosing and managing depression in the context of HIV disease. The severity of Juan's symptoms mandates intervention. But which interventions are best? Juan has a history of major depressive disorder severe enough to have warranted hospitalization, so he is clearly at risk for a recurrence. But a number of confounding variables muddle the clinical picture, not the least of which is Juan's advanced HIV disease and deteriorated immune system, which suggest that he is at risk for opportunistic infections of the central nervous system. These "organic" roots would require expeditious biological intervention such as antibiotics or chemotherapy. Likewise, Juan's cognitive difficulties, psychomotor slowness, and poor concentration could be explained by HIV-associated dementia. Dementia, with its characteristic apathy and lack of motivation, can easily be mistaken for depression. Juan's history of alcohol abuse could also cause cognitive decline and an alcohol-induced mood disorder. None of these etiological factors is mutually exclusive: Juan could have early cognitive impairment due to a combination of HIV and past alcohol abuse; he might be drinking currently and have an underlying recurrent major depression.

Beyond the more acute questions about medical etiology, Juan's case is complicated by important cultural and psychological concerns. Juan is an immigrant whose early upbringing occurred in another culture, and his first language is not English. He is not necessarily operating with the same values and expectations as the "average" American. In addition to these cross-cultural issues, Juan reports a relatively recent relationship breakup, and it was the end of a previous relationship that first sent Juan into crisis years before. In fact, a depressive reaction is an expected and healthy response to the breakup of a romantic relationship; how much might this contribute to Juan's current symptoms? Juan's response may also be influenced by characterological issues related to abandonment or separation.

Juan's psychiatrist consulted Juan's primary care physician to rule out major central nervous system (CNS) pathologies, referred Juan to a psychologist for neuropsychiatric testing to help rule out dementia, and confirmed Juan's sustained sobriety. Juan's psychiatrist then made a working diagnosis of recurrent major depression, but retained HIV-related dementia as a possible diagnosis that had to be ruled out. Because of a time lag of several weeks in obtaining neuropsychological testing results, the psychiatrist considered a trial of psychostimulant medication – which would have the advantage of addressing both dementia and depression – but he ultimately opted for an antidepressant trial, using the agent that had been effective during Juan's previous psychiatric hospitalization. Over the following few weeks, Juan's mental status improved dramatically. Neuropsychological testing uncovered prominent depression and mild cognitive deficits probably secondary to both HIV disease and Juan's history of alcohol use.

Juan also began psychotherapy, which provided him with support and helped him develop coping skills, and he saw a case manager to help with his social service needs. As Juan became more self-reliant, his psychotherapist changed the emphasis of therapy from structuring activities to engaging in a more psychodynamic process. Juan revealed that he had been inconsistent at the medical clinic because he perceived his primary care physician as "a busy American who didn't really care." When rejection came at the hands of "Americans," it set off profound feelings in Juan of inadequacy and self-denigration, typically with racial overtones. These deprecatory self-images were further supported by painful experiences of racial discrimination and poverty. At the medical clinic Juan attended, very few staff people spoke Spanish, and Juan often felt dismissed as an outsider who did not really belong there. Adherence and medical compliance were thus hampered by fundamental questions of trust, fueled by cultural tensions.

In therapy, Juan embarked on an exploration into the relationships among his sexuality, "Latino-ness," immigration, and past psychological traumas. Juan realized that he sometimes erroneously conceived of his HIV as a confirmation of his unworthiness, a revelation facilitated by his antidepressant regimen, which bolstered his internal reserve and his resiliency. Equipped with this understanding, Juan improved his alliance with his medical provider and began an HIV antiviral treatment regimen. His therapist also referred Juan to a support group for Latino gay men, which helped him consolidate the gains made in individual therapy and provided a greater sense of connection to his community.

Within six months, Juan was functioning well enough to fully care for himself. His CD4+ cell count had risen well above 200, and hospice care was neither appropriate nor necessary. With the help of his case manager, Juan successfully moved to independent housing and continued both antidepressant treatment and psychotherapy.

Facilitating a Biopsychosocial Approach

Obviously, not all cases of depression end with such dramatically positive results. But this case demonstrates that an approach to depression that carefully evaluates presenting symptoms and situates them in a truly biopsychosocial context can have a profound impact. Treatment strategies must be multifaceted, addressing the complex and interrelated needs of the individual. For Juan, this included stabilization with antidepressant medications in the context of a residential setting that could guarantee safety and close follow-up. But these interventions might not have been sufficient. The purpose of antidepressant medications was not simply to help rid Juan of his sadness and despair, but rather to facilitate his work in psychotherapy. In therapy, it was important that Juan experience a host of negative emotions: sadness about past and current losses, anger about perceived mistreatment and discrimination, and frustration about the daily nuisances of medication regimens. Without medication support these feelings might well have been overwhelming. It was psychotherapy that led to an understanding of Juan's disengagement from treatment a year earlier and his more general social isolation. Therapy helped clarify the relationship between Juan's history as an immigrant and his sense of being an "outsider," between his internalized homophobia and racism and his actual traumatic experiences of oppression and discrimination. Similarly, Juan's support group provided an environment in which Juan could further develop his sense of connectedness with others.

The approach advocated here often calls for a coordinated multidisciplinary team, particularly for clients who are the most disadvantaged, whether because of advanced physical decline, severe mental illness, or socioeconomic deprivation. When working with these individuals, the treatment team may have an especially important function as a stabilizing and integrative force. Ideally, mental health and social service components work in tandem with medical care, using open communication and extensive treatment coordination to ensure that treatment interventions at all levels work against the inherently disruptive forces of HIV disease and in favor of the best interests of the client.

Conclusion

Clinicians working with people with HIV disease should expect to see depressive symptoms in their clients, recognizing that expressions of distress are ubiquitous. Feelings of sadness are healthy and necessary expressions in the process of mourning the radical loss occasioned by HIV disease. But clinicians must also have a high index of suspicion for clinical levels of depression among their clients. While the literature on prevalence is not definitive, there is indication that increased HIV symptom profiles may put individuals at higher risk of clinical depression than people without HIV. Because clients and providers alike often inappropriately normalize depressive feelings, it is likely that clinical depression is undertreated in this population.

Genetic or acquired biological predispositions for depression unfold in the context of an individual's psychology and social relations, both of which may heighten or diminish the likelihood of clinical depression. In order to be effective, clinicians must formulate the depressive problem along biological, psychological, and sociocultural lines, and apply treatments in the context of a strong working alliance among a client's medical, psychiatric, psychotherapeutic, and social service providers. Failure to do so can result in truncated assessments, dehumanization, and short-sighted treatment strategies. Chapter Two deepens this overview by more closely examining variables in the biological, psychological, and sociocultural contexts specific to HIV-related depression.

2

The Context of Depression

To assess a client for the signs and symptoms of depression, a clinician must sift through an enormous amount of complicated evidence in search of a reasonable hypothesis about the root of the client's symptoms. The obvious goal of such a diagnostic process is the conceptualization of the problem in such a way that the clinician can formulate helpful interventions. As is clear from Chapter One, understanding the biopsychosocial "surround" of depression can lead to a more nuanced assessment strategy than can a symptom checklist alone. This chapter further explores this surround by examining specific variables, such as social stigma, coping style, and fatigue, and their particular relationship to HIV-associated depression, as well as a more detailed exploration of the subpopulations most affected by the epidemic.

The Biological Environment:
Depression in the Medically Ill

Diagnosing depression in the context of chronic medical illness has long been a problem for clinicians. As already noted, research to determine prevalence rates of clinical depression has been confounded by the equivocation of somatic and emotional symptoms. Indeed, weight loss, fatigue, and insomnia are hallmark features of clinical depression, but can also be common symptoms of medical illness and, in particular, of HIV disease. Similarly, malaise and poor energy due to physical illness can mimic a depressed mood or anhedonia, the inability to experience pleasure.

A number of studies in the late 1980s and early 1990s demonstrated a correlation between depression scores and HIV disease symptomatology. The Multicenter AIDS Cohort Study (MACS), based on a cohort of almost 5,000 homosexual men, found a clear association between depression ratings and self-report of HIV-related symptoms such as swollen lymph nodes, weight loss, and fever. [23] MACS subjects who had high HIV symptom levels scored twice as high on the measurement of somatic depression as subjects with lower HIV symptom levels.[15] Another study found that depressed subjects reported twice as many physical symptoms of HIV as non-depressed subjects.[24]

Consultation-liaison psychiatrists, who provide psychiatric consultation and management of medical patients, have long struggled with the question of how to diagnose depression in the medically ill. That there is overlap between medical illness symptoms and somatic depressive symptoms is generally acknowledged; the extent to which this overlap may confound a diagnosis of depression is a more controversial question. Some commentators argue that higher levels of depression predispose clients to a greater focus inward on to the physical and, in this way, to more somatic complaints. Others state that there is a confusing overlap between somatic symptoms of depression and medical illness, for example, when a report of physical fatigue is erroneously interpreted as lack of motivation. Still others contend that while somatic symptoms may cause some confusion, they ultimately do not confound the diagnosis of depression, because medically ill depressed clients usually exhibit sufficient psychological symptoms.[25]

While a clinician must ultimately work with a client as a whole person rather than as a constellation of symptoms, it is useful to review specific physical factors clinicians should consider in making a diagnosis of clinical depression among clients with HIV. Recognizing confounding medical variables such as fatigue, insomnia, and cognitive impairment is particularly important because they may be signs of other treatable conditions.

Fatigue and Insomnia

One of the most common and perplexing of the confounding variables is fatigue. Fatigue can mimic the complaints of low energy or poor motivation often found in those individuals with depressive disorders, and as might be expected is associated with later stage HIV disease, other AIDS-related physical symptoms, antiviral treatment for HIV-related medical disorders, and any HIV-related pain.[26] A study comparing HIV-negative and HIV-positive gay and bisexual men found that 14 percent of men with CD4+ cell counts of less than 500 suffered clinical fatigue.[27] While fatigue was more prominent in advanced HIV disease and was associated with depression, the study found that it did not seem simply to be a symptom of depression and could contribute independently to physical limitation and disability. A separate study found women were more likely to report fatigue than men.[26]

The etiology of fatigue is most likely multifactorial and varies from person to person. Malaise from HIV infection itself, opportunistic infections, or chronic diarrhea can all cause significant tiredness. Low serum testosterone levels or poor nutrition could also be offenders. Anemia may be caused directly by HIV or may be a side effect of some antiretroviral medications, most notably the now less commonly used zidovudine (ZDV; AZT): anemia produces low energy, shortness of breath on exertion, and headaches.

Insomnia may be a particularly important factor in producing fatigue, but must also be considered independently as a confounding variable of depression. In fact, high rates of sleep disturbance have been documented in people with HIV. In one review of 115 ambulatory persons with HIV (including mixed HIV transmission categories and various ethnicities), 73 percent of respondents qualified as having a sleep disturbance using the Pittsburgh Sleep Quality Index.[28] Cognitive impairment and depression were the best predictors of insomnia. As with fatigue, insomnia seems to be underrecognized: only 33 percent of the respondents with sleep disturbance had documentation of it in their medical record. Sleep problems seem to worsen with HIV disease progression, but also occur early in the disease before the development of other HIV-related symptoms. Some reports suggest that HIV infection of the brain may itself be responsible for initiating sleep disturbances by altering immune proteins that have a role in regulating sleep cycles.[29]

Despite the prevalence of fatigue among people with HIV disease, this factor is routinely underdiagnosed or unrecognized, perhaps because fatigue has long been considered an expected and untreatable condition of HIV illness. Increasingly, however, clinicians evaluate fatigue as an independent entity and recommend specific interventions for it. The first step is to develop a comprehensive differential diagnosis to determine the cause of fatigue, including, in addition to anxiety and depression, medication side effects, anemia, pain, infections or fever, hormonal or nutritional deficiency, inactivity, and sleep disturbance.[30]

Weight Loss

It is well-known that HIV can cause weight loss, and in clients with wasting syndrome, weight loss is the prominent symptom. In Africa, wasting is so common that AIDS is routinely referred to as "slim disease." Weight loss is more common in more advanced HIV disease than in earlier stage disease and is often accompanied by chronic diarrhea. With the broad use of protease inhibitors, clients and providers have also had to deal with lipodystrophy, a side effect that leads to the redistribution of fat stores in the body. While not an actual decrease in weight, lipodystrophy can reduce fat deposits in the cheeks or extremities, giving the appearance of weight loss.

Weight loss may complicate a diagnosis of clinical depression in two ways. As with lack of energy, weight loss is one of the diagnostic criteria for a DSM diagnosis of clinical depression, since individuals suffering from depression often manifest decreased appetite. Change in weight, real or apparent, can also operate as a mark of stigma, a physical manifestation of being sick that others can see. In this manner, weight loss can take on psychological meaning as an engine of depression in the psyche of the client.

Since its causes are manifold – including neoplasms, opportunistic infections, chronic diarrhea, and depression – diagnosing weight loss requires a thorough medical work-up. Most medical providers working with HIV aggressively investigate and treat weight loss in their patients, often prescribing appetite stimulators such as dronabinol.

Cognitive Impairment

Along with the symptoms of fatigue, insomnia, and weight loss, HIV can confound the assessment of clinical depression by its direct neurological effects. Many patients with HIV-associated dementia present with apathy, closely resembling anhedonia. Cognitive impairment may produce poor concentration, decreased interest, memory deficits, and psychomotor slowing that can be easily interpreted as the "pseudodementia" of depression. Theoretically, HIV could probably also directly cause organic depression through infection of the subcortex at sites that regulate emotion, though this has not been proven.

A controlled study comparing depressed and non-depressed HIV-infected men found that while depressed subjects performed less well on cognitive testing than non-depressed subjects, the majority of these men did not have significantly impaired memory, and there was no relationship between neuropsychological impairment and severity of depression.[31] The researchers conclude that while some HIV-infected men with depression perform more poorly on memory functions, they are not more likely to have clinically significant neurocognitive impairment. Indeed, studies have generally not found a clinically significant relationship between dementia and depression. Such results suggest that depression and dementia in HIV are clearly separable disorders. Because treatment approaches to these conditions can vary considerably, clinicians must make careful assessments to differentiate them.

The Psychosocial Environment: Coping and Support

The body may be the site of intense interactions – between immune proteins, viral particles, hormones, cells, and nameless other biochemical entities – but it is the mind that must represent the effects of these interactions and imbue them with meaning. An individual infected with HIV develops some way of understanding what is happening in his or her body and finds some way of dealing with it. The kinds of understanding and methods of coping are as varied as the individuals confronting this illness. Social science researchers have identified two sets of psychosocial variables that are important for understanding HIV-related depression: coping and social support.

Coping and the Locus of Control

"Coping styles" refers to the ways individuals react to and deal with stress. In the context of HIV disease, researchers have identified two major coping styles: active and passive.[32] In active coping, the individual directly confronts HIV-related stresses by obtaining information, investigating resources, and building a support network. These clients take charge of their own care: first by accepting the reality of what they are confronting, and second by employing a "fighting spirit" to maximize positive outcomes. Examples of active coping include seeking out services, confronting obstacles realistically, building a support network, volunteering, and expressing distress about stressful situations.

Individuals who use passive coping techniques, on the other hand, typically rely on avoiding sources of stress. These clients prefer not to think about HIV and use distraction or denial as a way of managing anxiety or depression. While some measure of denial is necessary and healthy to avoid being overwhelmed by the existential and at times catastrophic issues raised by HIV disease, passive coping can have significant negative consequences if employed as the mainstay against the HIV-related stress. Rather than seeking support for anxiety or depression, for example, such an individual may turn to alcohol or drugs to "forget." Avoidance can also promote poor adherence to medication regimens, which often serve as daily reminders of illness.

Whether a person employs active or passive styles of coping illustrates something about his or her assessment of "locus of control"; that is, it indicates what a client perceives as controllable, and by whom or what. Simplistically speaking, individuals who employ an active style of coping believe that they are able to influence outcomes and take charge of difficult situations. They tend to have realistic appraisals of what they are facing, be it medication side effects, treatment outcomes, or interpersonal difficulties. People who employ passive coping, on the other hand, locate control outside of themselves, believing that they cannot influence events. They tend to use denial and avoidance as ways of keeping anxieties at bay.

Active and passive coping styles are neither mutually exclusive nor monolithic; most individuals employ both. Further, while the passive style is often perceived as destructive or pathological, the truth is that denial is a necessary defense for everyone: an unremitting focus on the reality of inevitable death would be paralyzing for the most functional among us. In a similar way, an over-emphasis on control can serve as a pernicious, albeit effective, defensive strategy. Many things in life are simply not controllable, and in the face of this reality, the most appropriate response is to acknowledge the relative helplessness of the human condition through the expression of frustration, sadness, or anger. Burying these negative emotions by tenaciously holding onto fantasies of control may fuel clinically depressive states.

Clinicians must creatively struggle with this complexity: coping styles have variable utility for different clients in different contexts. When is it important for a client to feel sadness and grief rather than avoid these difficult emotions? When and how should a clinician motivate a client to act rather than to passively experience? When should a clinician challenge denial and when should he or she support it?

Social Support

A second important variable, and one that might be said to hover at the frontier between the psychological and the social, is social support. Fundamentally, social support describes the connectedness of an individual, that is, his or her sense of belonging to a social network. In the context of HIV, social support refers to the group of individuals on whom a client can rely to provide both practical and emotional assistance, including everything from helping with grocery shopping and laundry to talking about the difficulties of living with HIV. Interestingly, studies of social support do not typically measure how socially connected an individual actually is. Rather, they often rely on the subject's *perception* of support, indicating that, at least in part, the variable is psychological: the feeling of being connected, of being a part of a larger group, and of being sustained by that group may be as important as receiving the actual help itself.

A number of early studies found a relationship between perceived social support and lower rates of depression in HIV-positive individuals.[33-36] In one study, satisfaction with three kinds of social support – emotional, practical, and informational – was inversely correlated with depression both at the time of initial assessment and one year later.[33] In this sample of gay urban men, support was especially important for individuals experiencing symptoms; it served as a way to "gain a realistic perspective of their situation and develop effective coping strategies." In this way social support and coping strategies may be related. Hearing what others think may help bolster a realistic appraisal of difficult situations and promote active engagement rather than passive withdrawal. Certainly developing a network of people on whom one can rely is itself a strategy for active coping.

Social support may help mitigate depression by counteracting the effects of triggers and stressors that wear down an individual's healthy defenses. If one of the causes of depression is that an individual's capacity to bear adversity becomes overwhelmed, social support may extend that capacity, making individuals more resilient. A load shared is easier to bear. To act as such a buffer, however, social support must obviously provide resources that match the demands posed by the stressor.[37] Having coffee with a friend once a week is not going to be very helpful if a person's major stressor is that fatigue has made running the household nearly impossible. If coping style is an individual's most personal and immediate response to the biological threats and demands of HIV, then appropriate social support might be seen as one of the fueling stations that helps the individual remain active and engaged, steadily confronting the many challenges of HIV disease and, for that matter, depression. Beyond the close circle of friends and supporters, however, are diffuse but powerful social and cultural currents.

The Sociocultural Environment

Depression always unfolds in a particular sociocultural arena. These cultural environments affect an individual's response to events, the occurrence of psychiatric disorders, and the clinician's understanding of these disorders. The lexicon for the expression of symptoms is taken from a larger cultural dictionary, just as the specific words we use in communicating with one another are drawn from the larger storehouse of language. Likewise, social networks themselves take on the shape and idiom of the cultures that infuse them.

Culture is the foundation of social interactions: the undergirding paradigm of values, language, and gestures; the acceptable means of approach and proximity; the boundaries of a social encounter. This cultural matrix is not one more added element in the complexity of interactions; it is more like the soup in which these interactions stew. For most people, culture is invisible until they find themselves face to face with a culture different from their own. The phenomenon of culture may be most evident for clinicians in the United States when working with non-English-speaking immigrants from rural Latin America or Asia. However, cultural issues are at work in the daily encounters of clinical practice. An African American woman reared in the inner city will communicate her subjective distress using a different idiom than an urban gay man who is into circuit parties. A thorough understanding of depressive symptomatol-ogy must be attuned to these sociocultural subtleties.

Cross-cultural mental health practice has made it clear that depres-sion can present in different ways depending on the cultural milieu. In many traditional, less industrialized cultures, for example, depression can manifest more somatically than it does in the developed world. In these cases, symptoms may include headache, fatigue, temperature sen-sation, dizziness, or numbness. Presumably these cultures make a less marked distinction between mind and body, accounting for the greater fluidity of symptomatic expression. A man from rural Guatemala who reports sex with other men might not initially complain of sadness, but rather of weakness, trouble sleeping, and a hot "current" along the side of his face. Only a careful history and sufficient cultural knowledge will reveal a clinical depression that might respond to antidepressant treat-ment. Nor is the matter limited to symptoms of depression. The thera-peutic alliance could be damaged by a simple cultural misunderstand-ing when a clinician questions this client's insistence that he is neither gay nor bisexual, but rather "un hombre," since urban gay identity will mean little to this man who constructs his sense of self more around the sexual role he plays in an encounter than on the sex of his partner.

But whether in Latin America or Chicago, culture is not something exotic. It is always operative in a clinical encounter. Hospitals, clinics, cities, parts of the country, disciplines, races, genders, ethnic and reli-gious groups all have cultures that influence what occurs between client and provider. The culture of medicine may tragically misread the injection-drug user addicted to opiates and deny him morphine when he is in pain. A culture of bravado may insist that men externalize their depressive feelings of loss in thrill-seeking, alcohol, or violence, rather than in intimate tearful moments. Wearing black and crying daily for two weeks may be a healthy response to grief in one culture and a symptom of a clinical disorder in another. Clinicians must recognize that culture exerts an influence on the clinical encounter and that symptoms can best be interpreted in the light of cultural contexts.

To best understand the issues that particular cultures face, it is use-ful to review depression prevalence studies for subpopulations of peo-ple with HIV. These studies offer not only a portrait of the epidemiology of clinical depression and HIV, but also an overview of the sociocultural factors that influence the prevalence and expression of depression and how these elements interact with medical and psychological factors.

Gay and Bisexual Men

Most controlled studies using standardized measures of depression have been conducted with samples of largely White, middle class, gay and bisexual men in the United States.[38-41] Rates of clinical depression in these cohorts range from around 6 percent to almost 50 percent. What is common across these studies is the finding of high lifetime rates of depressive and substance abuse disorders, as high as 30 percent to 50 percent of the samples for both disorders. But evidence that these disorders often precede HIV infection and that their rates are significantly higher than rates in heterosexual control groups indicates that being gay or bisexual, rather than HIV-positive, may be most salient.

Probably the best explanation for the high rates of depression among gay and bisexual men is that homosexuality remains deeply stigmatized. While this is clearly changing, most HIV-positive gay men did not experience social acceptance during childhood and adolescence. Stigma operates not only as a social force – in the form of discrimination and violence – but also more subtley as a psychological one. Gay children still are seldom recognized as such by their families, friends, and teachers, growing up without acknowledgment of vital parts of their identity. Some gay men develop a "closet psychology," in which aspects of themselves, particularly sexual ones, remain disconnected from the fabric of their lives. Social restrictions reinforce this tendency.

Further, clinical practice indicates that a number of seropositive gay men harbor conscious or unconscious guilt about their HIV infection, which they sometimes see as punishment for social or sexual "transgressions." After fifteen years of ubiquitous safer sex campaigns in urban gay communities, individuals who have recently seroconverted may feel even guiltier about having done so. HIV can replicate the stigmatized social structure of being gay: it sets up another division between public and private, acceptance and rejection, normal and ill.

One of the biggest differences between straight and queer culture is the role and function of sex. A celebratory stance towards sexuality has been a hallmark of gay freedom movements, and urban gay men continue to have easy access to recreational sex. The uses of gay sex – as consolidator of identity, joyful expression, means of managing anxiety or loneliness, search for love and connection – are as varied as the men who practice it. HIV becomes a powerful symbol in this sexual landscape: a marker of stigma, isolation, shame, punishment, or defiance.

The converse of homophobic stigma, at least in some gay urban centers of the United States, has been the development of an HIV community. Today, there is a vast array of HIV services forged in the crucible of gay and lesbian culture, and gay and bisexual men usually do not have to cross a cultural divide to obtain quality HIV services in the major cities. This kind of culturally syntonic support may provide some measure of protection against depression for some individuals. WHO researcher Mario Maj has speculated that the lack of a difference in prevalence rates for clinical depression between HIV-positive and HIV-negative gay men in the United States is due to the protective effects of this social support among HIV-positive men, who, in fact, may have more social support than their HIV-negative counterparts.[42]

Women

In the United States, women represent one of the fastest growing groups of people with HIV disease. The majority of women with HIV were either infected via injection drug use or through heterosexual sex with an infected partner (who himself has been infected either through sex with men or via injection drug use). Because some of the most dramatic increases in HIV infection rates for women have been in communities of color, particularly Latina and African American women, studies describing depression rates among women often include high representation from these groups.

Several recent studies of HIV-infected women have found rates of clinically significant depression of almost 50 percent. In a multiethnic study done at Cook County Hospital in Chicago, chart review revealed that 47 percent of the 193 women seen in an HIV specialty program had signs of depression.[3] In another multiethnic sample of 53 women with HIV, 40 percent had clinically significant rates of depressive symptomatology and anxiety.[44] In a Pittsburgh study of 36 HIV-positive women at a primary care practice, lifetime prevalence rates were 49 percent for major depression and 9 percent for dysthymia.[45]

As is true in studies of gay and bisexual men, while these are remarkably high rates, the relative significance of the numbers remains a matter of interpretation. In the Pittsburgh study, for instance, rates for depression and dysthymia for HIV-positive women were similar to those of socioeconomically matched HIV-negative women, consistent with an earlier study.[46] Other studies, however, have found rates of depression to increase with HIV infection: for example, one study found higher mean depressive scores in African American, Puerto Rican, and non-Hispanic White HIV-infected women than in normative samples.[47] It is difficult to compare some of these studies because they use different time criteria to define prevalence.

Each of these studies highlights questions of access to care. In the Cook County study, for example, of the 90 women with documented depression, only 74 percent received some sort of treatment for depression: 36 percent received antidepressants and 66 percent received mental health counseling. In the Pittsburgh study, fully half of the women meeting criteria for a DSM diagnosis of depression had not sought out professional help. Both of these studies were conducted in primary care settings where it might be expected that patients could be appropriately referred to mental health providers with relative ease. Other researchers have noted that despite the efficacy of treatment for depression in women, treatment attrition rates can be high because the unmet psychosocial needs of clients may interfere with treatment adherence.[48]

Recognition of women's needs came to be understood relatively late in the epidemic, so that research on depression in HIV-positive women and resources for their care remained inadequate until recently. The mental health needs of women are notably different from those of gay and bisexual men. Unlike gay men, many women do not consider themselves at risk for HIV, and there is relatively little consciousness in many women's social networks about HIV-related risk factors. As a result, a heterosexual woman may feel doubly betrayed when she simultaneously discovers she is seropositive and that her male partner is either having sex with men or injecting drugs. If she becomes pregnant, she must further deal with issues about whether to have the child; child care itself constitutes an additional psychological and economic burden, particularly if the child is also HIV-infected.

Women are particularly vulnerable to social stigma.[49] Many women infected with HIV are women of color, and thus carry a triple risk for discrimination: gender, race or ethnicity, and HIV serostatus. Additionally, women with HIV are often poor, caring for dependent children as single heads of household,[50] and must contend with the general socioeconomic gender disparity in the United States.

Finally, physical or sexual trauma forms a prominent part of the mental health picture for many women. Depression among women has been significantly associated with a history of physical and sexual abuse, while post-traumatic symptoms have been associated with increased HIV-related risk taking.[51,52] Even in the absence of blatant abuse, emotional or economic coercion may be a subtle but pernicious component of sexual exchanges. In the context of physical or sexual trauma, HIV infection – itself a traumatic event – can aggravate feelings of helplessness, anger, self-blame, or guilt. All of these emotional challenges can be further complicated by isolation, putting some women at higher risk for depression. In both urban and rural communities, women may find themselves alone with few social supports.[53] The epidemic among women – unlike among gay men – is often shrouded in silence, and women may avoid disclosing to family or friends.[54]

Injection Drug Users

Studies of injection drug users show the same variation in prevalence rates as studies of gay and bisexual men and women. Some studies have found higher rates of current depressive disorders such as major depression and dysthymia among seropositive subjects: about 33 percent for HIV-positive and 15 percent for HIV-negative drug using individuals.[55,56] Other studies have not found significant difference in depression rates on the basis of serostatus.[57,58] But, even studies that have not found different rates of depression have documented higher levels of depression for injection drug users than for people in the general population. Again, the fundamental question regarding prevalence data is: are higher depression rates attributable to HIV status *per se* or to issues related to injection drug use? Several variables help to interpret these prevalence studies and begin to answer this question.

First, depression in injection drug users is correlated with higher rates of drug use and of HIV-related risk behavior such as using unclean needles or sharing needles.[59-62] Drug use can be seen as the epitome of avoidant behavior, that is, passive coping, which as noted earlier, can lead to a greater vulnerability to depressive symptoms. While HIV seroconversion motivates sobriety in many substance users, it is common to hear drug-using clients report that they have dramatically increased their use after seroconversion, usually as a way to deal with anxiety and depression. HIV infection can initiate a negative feedback loop, in which infection is seen as confirmation of low self-esteem and worthlessness, which leads to greater drug use as a way of extinguishing these intolerable emotions. In addition, by prompting higher risk behaviors such as needle sharing, depression may also promote the spread of HIV by weakening the resolve of injection drug users to protect others.

Second, female injection drug users have higher rates of depression than male users.[63,64] Risk factors for depression among women in these studies include lower self-esteem, low economic status, and greater numbers of sex partners. As noted above, women face discrimination, economic disadvantage, and power differences that might be internalized as poor self-esteem, turning an external disparity into a psychological handicap. The correlation between depression and a greater number of sex partners may also relate to another potential risk factor: sexual or physical trauma. Clinical experience underscores the frequency with which sexual trauma surfaces as the root of a multidimensional psychiatric problem, often preceding and contributing to drug use and HIV risk. Finally, as is true for other populations, both male and female drug users benefit from social support.[55]

People of Color

Very little has been written comparing the prevalence rates of depression in communities of color to other subgroups or the general population. As noted above, a number of studies of women and drug users include large proportions of African Americans and Latinos, but the overall numbers are usually too small to result in meaningful intergroup comparisons. There is virtually no specific literature on depression in Native American or Asian/Pacific Islander American groups, both of which include small numbers of HIV-infected individuals.

There is a much more substantial literature on HIV prevention for Latinos and African Americans, but there is little on the diagnosis and treatment of psychiatric disorders in these communities. This lack of data partly reflects the realities of the epidemic: there is a great deal of overlap among risk groups, and for epidemiological reasons, study subjects are usually categorized according to the behaviors that led to infection. While studies by transmission risk still uncover data relevant to communities of color, it is drug use and sexual transmission, rather than race and ethnicity, that become the dominant frames of analysis. The paucity of literature on communities of color also reflects the more insidious and stubborn problems of invisibility, structural discrimination, and lack of resources faced by these communities.

The literature on HIV prevention in women and in gay and bisexual men of color suggests that social disadvantage and disempowerment may contribute to an increased risk of becoming infected.[65] It stands to reason that these sociocultural factors remain operative once an individual becomes infected and thus could affect the development of depressive symptoms. Indeed, stigmatized groups always face uphill battles in the struggle for recognition and legitimacy. Having to deal with the multiple stigmatizing forces of HIV serostatus, race, gender, sexual orientation, and drug use could naturally erode the psychosocial resources that might help prevent depression. In a study of perceived control regarding health care, seropositive African American and Latino subjects were significantly more likely than seropositive White subjects to believe their health status was in the hands of powerful others or of chance.[66] Such views correlated with greater psychological difficulty. It is notable that women and subjects of lower socioeconomic status were more likely to report this externalized locus of control.

Several studies have documented the role of social stressors on the development of psychological difficulties in HIV-positive African Americans. A study of African American men of all sexual orientations demonstrated no significant differences with respect to HIV serostatus on measures of depression, but noted that psychosocial resources mediated the effect of stressors on mood.[67] A 1994 study of homosexually active African American men and women hypothesized that these individuals might be at higher risk of psychiatric dysfunction due to their multiple stigmatized social statuses.[68] The study found that African American women who had sex with women were as distressed as HIV-infected gay African American men. Both men and women in this study reported higher levels of distress than the general population of African Americans or White gay and bisexual men.

Hopelessness and the Evolution of Stigma

The history of the epidemic has created a culture of HIV that affects people with HIV who belong to all subpopulations. A key factor in this history is the stigmatization and isolation of people with HIV, which unfolded for a variety of reasons, including: the panic that followed the emergence of AIDS, the lack of information about its etiology and nature, the absence of cure or treatment, and the focus of the epidemic on marginalized groups, in particular, gay and bisexual men and injection drug users.[69,70] This stigmatization warped public policy, leading to an inadequate public health response that further fanned fear and created suffering. Ironically, marginalization ultimately fostered a grassroots activist response, an active coping mechanism that led to significant change and actually reduced stigma as well as improved services.

This history of stigma is long from forgotten and continues to influence even newly infected people with HIV. For many, HIV infection only compounds the already heavy social taboos of homosexuality, race, gender, or injection drug use. For others, HIV infection alone is enough to provoke the animosity and violence of others. The effects of such cultural branding operate on both social and psychological levels. Around some people, stigma draws an estranging curtain of silence, effectively separating them from their network of social support. While extensive education and public health campaigns have made this less likely in White urban gay communities, stigma remains a palpable force in rural areas, among some heterosexuals, and in communities of color – in any social sphere, that is, where the epidemic is not publicly embraced. As an internalized force, stigma can also be a devastating blow to the psyche: it is an endlessly renewable source of self-deprecation, all too easily corroborated by everyday realities. Social marginalization hampers social support networks, decreases access to services, increases victimization, and reduces self-esteem, all of which compromise resilience and increase vulnerability to depressive symptoms.

Conclusion

A number of variables influence the development of clinical depression in the context of HIV. While these may confound research, they suggest valuable areas of investigation in the clinical setting, offering useful information for assessment and treatment planning. For example, medical variables such as fatigue, insomnia, and cognitive impairment may complicate the diagnosis of depression, but they may also provide direction for clinicians designing interventions. Identifying a client's coping styles, both passive and active, may provide important clues to his or her psychotherapeutic needs and ability to adhere to medication regimens. Finally, clients with HIV are often members of groups that have experienced extraordinary discrimination. The impact of such marginalization is apparent in limited access to care and inadequate care systems, in debilitated social networks, and in internalized stigma. Understanding the social and cultural significance of HIV is an important route to understanding marginalization and the value of social support as a protective factor against depression. Chapter Three considers the formal assessment of clinical depression, a task that can be undertaken only with sensitivity to the broader range of biopsychosocial factors presented in this chapter.

3

Assessing Depression

Perhaps the most difficult challenge facing clinicians assessing depression is to distinguish between the expected and healthy expression of sadness over loss, which is unavoidable in people with HIV, and the clinical syndrome of depression, whose symptoms significantly interfere with day-to-day functioning. This chapter focuses on these challenges in clinical assessment, outlining a method for diagnosing depressive illness that applies standard psychiatric approaches while integrating principles derived from the biopsychosocial analysis outlined in Chapter Two. At the core of the chapter is a thorough understanding of major depressive disorder, the archetype of depressive illness, whose major symptoms are common to many other forms of depression. The chapter examines the processes both for conducting an assessment and for differentiating major depression from other depressive illnesses. It begins with the role of front-line providers who, as frequent sources of referral to mental health professionals, serve as preliminary screeners of depression and crucial channels to treatment.

The Role of Front-Line Providers

While mental health clinicians will probably ultimately become involved in the diagnosis and management of clients with clinical depressions, both social service staff (including case managers, treatment and peer advocates, and other non-mental health staff) and medical personnel play a vital role in the treatment process of depression. Because depressive symptoms are so common among HIV-positive individuals, and because they can have such a significant impact both on a client's quality of life and his or her ability to care for him or herself, social service providers should be vigilant for symptoms and be prepared to refer clients for evaluation. Initiating a dialogue with the client is probably the single most effective intervention at this point. Social service providers should acknowledge to the client the symptoms he or she has noted – for example, sadness, poor motivation, tearfulness, or fatigue – and talk about how lasting or serious these have been. In general, providers who find themselves worrying about a client's well-being should probably refer the client for further evaluation.

Primary care providers are often the first health care professionals to identify symptoms of depression among patients. They are well-advised to screen all clients with HIV for clinical depression by following two steps. First, since a history of clinical depression is among the strongest predictors of future recurrence, historical information can provide a sense of the severity and frequency of past clinical depressive episodes, and can alert the clinician to the intensity of monitoring required in the future. At a minimum, this history should include a record of past hospitalizations and medication trials for depression as well as questions about past suicidal intention or actual suicide attempts. If there were attempts, the clinician should note the means, whether medical intervention was necessary, medical and psychiatric responses to the attempt, and the client's reaction to the attempt.

Second, practitioners should follow-up by routinely inquiring about mood symptoms during the period prior to appointments. Simple and direct questions – How has your mood been recently? Do you ever feel depressed or sad? – can suggest whether more in-depth inquiries are necessary. If there is evidence of current depressive distress, practitioners should evaluate clients using standard DSM-IV criteria (see below).

It bears repeating that not all individuals will demonstrate "classic" depressive symptoms, and "externalizing" behaviors such as drug use, violence, and sexual promiscuity may be the most prominent features of depression. Further, cultural manifestations can alter the presentation of depression; for example as mentioned in Chapter Two, emotional symptoms may manifest as bodily complaints. Primary care providers should also consider more in-depth evaluation for patients who are having trouble adhering to HIV-related medical treatment, since poor adherence has been correlated with depression.[71]

Front-line providers should be guided by three principles when screening for depression: duration, severity, and undertreatment. Healthy expressions of sadness or depression are transient: they should not become a way of life, and more than two weeks of depressive symptoms should raise clinical suspicions. Even if transient, the severity of a response, most obviously, acute suicidality, should demand further intervention. If the severity of symptoms puts the client or others at significant risk of harm or severely interrupts functioning, the provider should refer the client for evaluation. Finally, depression in the context of HIV is common and too often undertreated, and referral for further assessment is, for all practical purposes, risk-free. A consultation with a mental health provider might help capture these overlooked cases.

The Core Symptoms of Major Depression

Psychiatric diagnoses establish a clear dividing line between healthy expressions of psychological distress and the impairing symptoms of a functional disorder. They serve as tools to help organize complex phenomena and, more importantly, to help plan interventions. The major compendium of psychiatric diagnoses is, of course, the DSM-IV, which uses functional impairment as the essential indicator of a clinical disorder. In this context, the DSM-IV description of a Major Depressive Episode is the cornerstone for diagnosing clinical depression. The criteria for a major depressive episode (see Table 1: Diagnostic Criteria for a Major Depressive Episode) represent an attempt to standardize or objectify symptoms, which is critical not only for clinical work, but also for the research that makes evidence-based interventions possible.

At the heart of the diagnosis of major depression is a depressed mood or the loss of pleasure (also known as "anhedonia") lasting at least two weeks. The term "depression" has a wide variety of meanings, so in investigating these symptoms, it is useful to ask clients to describe their moods in some detail. Open-ended questions (rather than yes/no questions) provide much more detailed and useful information. Consider questions such as:

◆ What do you mean when you say "depression" (or "anxiety" or "feeling down," for example)?

◆ Describe this feeling.

◆ Do you cry? How often? What do you cry about?

◆ Dealing with HIV is usually very difficult. How do you cope when things get rough?

In assessing for anhedonia, in particular, ask: What kinds of things do you enjoy? Most clinically depressed individuals will have difficulty providing a convincing answer, and the clinician can then follow up with more specific inquiries.

Having established a history of depressive mood or anhedonia, the clinician then attempts to amass evidence for other principle symptoms. Besides depressed mood or anhedonia, clients must demonstrate at least four out of an additional seven symptoms drawn from the DSM-IV checklist in order to qualify for a diagnosis of major depression. The first four of these additional symptoms can be said to occur at the frontier between mind and body and are often termed "vegetative" or somatic symptoms. These include sleep and appetite disturbances, fatigue, and psychomotor speed (background body movements, like nervous fidgeting or sluggishness). As much as possible, clinicians should attempt to quantify changes in weight (pounds lost or gained in last month, for example) and sleep changes (note regular times for going to bed and getting up, time it takes to fall asleep, total estimated hours slept in a typical night). These somatic symptoms can complicate the evaluation of depression in the context of HIV, since physical illness can produce similar effects. Difficulty concentrating or indecision is another somatic symptom, which can manifest as memory or problem-solving difficulties.

The remaining symptoms of clinical depression are solidly affective, that is, relating to emotion. These include feelings of guilt or worthlessness, moribund thinking (thoughts of death), or frank suicidality. Unlike the vegetative signs, these symptoms are clearly indicative of depression, since they are not confounded by physical illness. As with the assessment for depressive mood or anhedonia, it is useful to use broad, open-ended questions here to obtain an in-depth view of the client's relationship to him or herself.

Table 1. Diagnostic Criteria for a Major Depressive Episode

Reprinted with permission from: American Psychiatric Association. Diagnostic and Statistical Manual of Mental Disorders, Fourth Edition. *Washington, D.C.: American Psychiatric Association, 1994. Copyright 1994 American Psychiatric Association.*

A. Five (or more) of the following symptoms have been present during the same two-week period and represent a change from previous functioning; at least one of the symptoms is either (1) depressed mood or (2) loss of interest or pleasure.

  1. Depressed mood most of the day, nearly every day, as indicated by either subjective report (for example, feels sad or empty) or observation made by others (for example, appears tearful).

  2. Markedly diminished interest or pleasure in all, or almost all, activities most of the day, nearly every day (as indicated by either subjective account or observation made by other).

  3. Significant weight loss when not dieting or weight gain (for example, a change of more than 5 percent of body weight in a month) or decrease or increase in appetite nearly every day.

  4. Insomnia or hypersomnia nearly every day.

  5. Psychomotor agitation or retardation nearly every day (observable by others, not merely subjective feelings of restlessness or being slowed down).

  6. Fatigue or loss of energy nearly every day.

  7. Feelings of worthlessness or excessive or inappropriate guilt (which may be delusional) nearly every day (not merely self-reproach or guilt about being sick).

  8. Diminished ability to think or concentrate, or indecisiveness, nearly every day (either by subjective account or as observed by others).

  9. Recurrent thoughts of death (not just fear of dying), recurrent suicidal ideation without specific plan, or a suicide attempt or a specific plan for committing suicide.

B. The symptoms do not meet criteria for a Mixed Episode.

C. The symptoms cause clinically significant distress or impairment in social, occupational, or other important areas of functioning.

D. The symptoms are not due to the direct physiological effects of a substance (for example, a drug of abuse, a medication) or a general medical condition (for example, hypothyroidism).

E. The symptoms are not better accounted for by bereavement, that is, after the loss of a loved one, and the symptoms persist for longer than two months or are characterized by marked functional impairment, morbid preoccupation with worthlessness, suicidal ideation, psychotic symptoms, or psychomotor retardation.

Major depression can be a life-threatening illness, and the assessment of suicidality deserves special attention. Clinicians should begin to assess suicidality by asking general questions, becoming gradually more specific. A good opening question is: Do things ever get so bad that you have thoughts of death or dying? Affirmative answers should prompt the provider to ask about details regarding the thoughts and fantasies, including their frequency and emotional quality. Having broached the subject of death, the interview can proceed specifically to suicidality: Do you ever have thoughts of harming yourself or of suicide? Any suicidal ideation should be explored in depth. The primary goal is to assess the risk of actual suicide. Clinicians should evaluate risk using five criteria: intention, planning, means, history, and impulsivity. Most people have probably had the idea of suicide at one time or another; thoughts, in and of themselves, are not dangerous. The real question is whether the individual has the intention to do harm to him or herself.

It can be helpful to make this distinction between thought or fantasy and action explicit to the client, and to ask how close he or she is to the "line" of action. Ideas of suicide usually take the form of specific ways of harm such as jumping off of a bridge or taking an overdose. The clinician should explore details of any plan mentioned by the client, and its specificity, for example, is the client considering overdose with a specific drug? Next, the provider should assess whether the client has the means to carry the plan to fruition. Does the client have the drugs at hand? How would he or she obtain them? Evaluation of the intent, plan, and means of suicide focuses on the current mental state of the client, but it is also valuable to consider past behavior. The clinician should review any history of suicide attempts in terms of planning, intention, means, precipitating factors, and the client's interpretations and reactions to the events. Finally, the clinician should consider if there are any aggravating circumstances that might compromise a client's judgment and make him or her more impulsive: for example, psychotic symptoms, the use of mind-altering drugs, the presence of dementia or delirium, or confusion from fever or medication effects.

The last four criteria for the diagnosis of a major depressive episode determine functional impairment and exclude other possible disorders. Regardless of the number of affective and vegetative symptoms present, a client will not meet criteria for major depression if these symptoms do not significantly impact his or her life. The exclusionary criteria listed in the DSM-IV definition for major depression rule out pre-existing substance abuse disorders, underlying medical conditions, and bipolar affective disorder (the "Mixed Episode" referred to in criteria B), as well as normal bereavement. The DSM-IV also recognizes two sub-types of major depression: single episode and recurrent. The recurrent variety is defined by the presence of two or more single episodes separated by at least two consecutive months.

Assessing Clinical History

A full exploration of a client's clinical history allows the provider to integrate biological, psychosocial, and cultural aspects, turning a flat snapshot of symptoms into a three-dimensional model, and helps determine the client's strengths and vulnerabilities. A careful history also facilitates the construction of a rigorous differential diagnosis. While a complete review of clinical history taking is beyond the scope of this monograph, three major areas are particularly pertinent to HIV-related depression: family, psychiatric, and psychosocial histories. In general, this assessment process should place clinical history and core symptoms of depression in the context of HIV illness (see Table 2: Checklist for the Assessment of HIV-Related Depression).

A history of psychiatric illness in the family provides evidence of a possible genetic predisposition toward depressive and other disorders, for example, psychosis or bipolar affective disorder. Family histories of psychiatric disorders are often obscure because of the stigma attached to mental illness. In response, the clinician should inquire about symptoms and other manifestations of clinical depression among family members (rather than simply asking about the disorders by name), including, for example, hospitalizations, use of antidepressant medication, and suicidal behaviors.

The family history may give some indication of the client's vulnerability to depressive illness, but the individual history provides a context through which to evaluate the current symptoms. One useful way to organize the individual psychiatric and psychosocial histories is with respect to HIV-related events, for instance, first diagnosis, development of symptoms, change in immune status, AIDS diagnosis, and initiation of antiviral treatment. HIV-related events are traumatic, requiring active accommodation and adjustment, and exploring how the client reacts to these events helps clarify his or her resilience and vulnerabilities, coping styles, and degree of social support. A good example is the reaction to an HIV diagnosis. Questioning can break down this process into its component psychological steps and reveal how the client manages the stress of HIV. How did the client learn of the diagnosis? Did the client take the initiative to test for HIV, or did others pressure him or her into it? How long did he or she wait to test after suspecting it might be necessary? What did the client expect the results would be and why? How did he or she react? Whom, if anyone, did he or she tell, and how did he or she make the decision to tell others?

Differentiating Depression from Other Conditions

After determining from an analysis of symptoms and family and clinical history that a client is suffering from depressive symptoms, the task is to rule out conditions other than major depressive disorder that would account for these symptoms. This process of "differential diagnosis" requires developing a comprehensive history, conducting a thorough mental status examination, obtaining information from outside sources such as service providers or family members when appropriate, and undertaking laboratory studies (sometimes including brain imaging) to rule out medical etiologies. The differential diagnosis for HIV-related depression can be divided into two major categories: primary and secondary depressions. Primary depressive disorders, sometimes referred to in the past as "functional" disorders, can be described as "endogenous," as having their origins "inside" the mind of the individual. Secondary depressive disorders, referred to in the past as "organic," are "exogenous," having their origins "outside" the individual, for example, as a result of substance abuse, medical conditions, or medication side effects. Most practitioners today would consider the distinction between "functional" and "organic" depressions to be archaic, if not fallacious. The very fact that pharmacology is effective in combating endogenous or functional depressions suggests that these disorders share an "organic" component. The distinction between primary and secondary seems more helpful and accurate.

A typical approach to constructing the differential diagnosis begins by ruling out secondary causes of a depression, whose treatment is vastly different from and sometimes more urgent than the treatment of primary causes. A client with psychomotor slowing and poor motivation might have a brain lesion requiring immediate attention, rather than major depression. Likewise, if depressive symptoms are due pri-

Table 2. Checklist for the Assessment of HIV-Related Depression

In addition to following routine assessment for depression, as suggested by the DSM-IV, clinicians should also review a range of HIV-related issues

HISTORY OF PRESENT ILLNESS

At what point in the progression of HIV disease does the individual present with depressive symptoms? What is the relationship of depression to the stage of the disease?

SEROCONVERSION

How and why did the individual decide to test for HIV? Had the client tested before? How often? Why? What did the individual anticipate would be the result? Why? How did the client react to the actual news of the results, including emotional, behavioral, and cognitive responses? How does the individual believe he or she became infected?

MEDICAL ISSUES

Does the client have an established relationship with a primary care provider? If not, why not? What is the client's current CD4+ count and viral load? What medical symptoms is the client experiencing, and what is his or her emotional response to these symptoms? Is there a history of opportunistic infections or major illnesses, especially CNS-related illness? What medications is the client taking? Is the client adhering to the medication regimen?

Check for "medical rule outs," which might confound a diagnosis of depression. Does the client suffer from fatigue, insomnia, or weight loss? Has there been a medical work-up of these symptoms?

SOCIAL SUPPORT

Who comprises the client's social support network, including family, friends, and support groups? How open is the individual about his or her serostatus? Who knows about his or her diagnosis?

MENTAL STATUS EXAM

Does the client need to be referred for cognitive assessment and neuropsychological testing?

marily to withdrawal from cocaine use, treatment should focus on issues related to substance use. After ruling out the secondary causes of depression, the differential diagnosis considers primary depressive disorders, including major depression (both unipolar and bipolar), dysthymia, and adjustment disorders. The diagnostic process also considers other major psychiatric disorders such as psychotic and anxiety disorders, and finally, personality disorders.

Substance-Induced Mood Disorders

An assessment of substance use should be part of any comprehensive psychiatric evaluation. For seropositive clients, such an evaluation is essential, since there are high rates of substance use in some of the groups at highest risk for becoming HIV infected. This is true not only in the obvious case of individuals who contracted HIV through injection drug use, but also among gay men, who have higher rates of substance use than the general population.[72]

Because substance use disorders are stigmatized in most cultures, it is crucial to have established a rapport with clients before attempting to inquire about a history of drug use, and to undertake this interview in a non-threatening, matter-of-fact way. It is often helpful to normalize drug use as a way of coping by saying, for example, that it is not unusual for people to use drugs or alcohol to deal with the stress of seroconversion. Empathy, rather than judgment, establishes the ground not only for an honest interchange but also for the treatment alliance.

An assessment of substance use should be specific and detailed. The clinician should ask about potential substances individually. For example, instead of asking, "Do you use any drugs?" ask "Do you ever use speed? marijuana? alcohol?" and so forth. Affirmative responses should prompt further inquiry to discover: duration and time frame of use; quantities used; triggers that encourage use; effects of use; reactions to withdrawal or discontinuation of use; the enjoyable aspects of the substance; and whether and why there were attempts to quit or reduce use. In assessing the contribution of substance use to the symptoms of depression, it is helpful first to take completely separate histories for substance use and mood, and then to correlate them in terms of timing with further input from the client. Thus, the provider might first ask about amphetamine use, and then separately obtain a detailed history about symptoms of depression. If there seems to be a correlation between the two, especially in terms of chronology, the provider can then suggest this correlation to the client. This same approach may be used to correlate HIV-related events with mood and substance use. Finally, any substance may be employed by the client as a means of escaping uncomfortable emotions or painful realities. The clinician should try to understand the role of the substance use in the client's life. This may provide clues to an underlying psychiatric disorder such as depression. Such passive coping in the form of "self-medication" can sustain an existing depression or erode the psychological skills needed to protect against a future depressive disorder.

Alcohol is almost certainly the most frequently abused substance and a common cause of depression. Among the other various substances, stimulants – particularly cocaine (including crack) and amphetamine – deserve special mention because they can easily mimic depressive symptoms. Depression due to stimulant withdrawal can be acute and severe, and can be further complicated by psychosis, which sometimes requires hospitalization. Stimulant use can also easily mimic bipolar affective disorder with its energetic highs and precipitous lows. Amphetamines have found a niche in gay men's culture as the fuel for the circuit party scene. Some gay men use amphetamines almost exclusively in the context of recreational sex, and uncovering this relationship can be an important part of assessment.

Marijuana use, though frequently encountered by HIV practitioners, is rarely the cause of depressive illness. Many HIV-positive patients use marijuana medicinally, to stimulate appetite or respond to the gastrointestinal side effects of medications. Dronabinol (Marinol), a medication with tetrahydrocannabinol (THC), the active substance in marijuana, is also routinely used for appetite stimulation in people with HIV-related wasting syndrome or weight loss. Some clients use both marijuana and Marinol concurrently, potentiating both the positive and negative effects. Regular marijuana use can produce severe apathy, which can mimic or exacerbate depressive symptoms. Because THC also suppresses rapid eye motion (REM) sleep, abrupt discontinuation of the substance in an individual who has been using it regularly produces "REM rebound," characterized by vivid dreaming and sleep disruption. Since sleep disruption is one of the vegetative signs of clinical depression, it is important to identify REM rebound as part of a differential diagnosis.

Jeremy: The Effects of Substance Use

Jeremy, a 32-year-old, African American, gay man was diagnosed with AIDS three months before complaining to his doctor that he was depressed. Since the diagnosis, Jeremy says he is feeling unmotivated and exhausted. He also says he feels suicidal "a lot." During these depressive crises, Jeremy usually stays at home in bed, isolated from his friends. After a few days, he is "more or less back to normal" and does not feel suicidal. Over the past few weeks, Jeremy has noted that he occasionally hears a voice whispering "You're no good," even when it is clear that he is alone. He has never been treated for depression before.

Jeremy's doctor initially suspected a diagnosis of major depression, perhaps with psychotic features, provoked by the stress of Jeremy's AIDS diagnosis. But as he began to take a substance use history, it became clear that Jeremy had used amphetamines "sometimes." After a more detailed history, Jeremy acknowledged that he had been using about a quarter gram of amphetamines, which he snorted, about every other weekend since the AIDS diagnosis. On "crashing," Jeremy usually also used marijuana. It was during these withdrawal periods that Jeremy felt depressed and suicidal. The whispering voice had frightened Jeremy enough that he sought help, but he felt ashamed about the drug use and was unable to volunteer the information.

Depression Induced by Medical Condition or Medications

According to the DSM-IV, depression due to a medical condition requires "evidence from the history, physical examination, or laboratory findings that the disturbance is the direct physiological consequence of a general medical condition."[13] Additionally, the diagnosis must exclude as the cause of such a disturbance another primary mental disorder, for example, adjustment disorder. If these criteria are met, and the depression causes significant impairment of function, then the DSM-IV recognizes two subtypes of this depression: mood disorder due to general medical condition with depressive features, and mood disorder due to general medical condition with major depressive-like episode. The difference between the two is the severity of symptoms, the second being more severe.

While HIV directly infects brain tissue,[73] there is no clear evidence that viral infection alone can cause clinical depression. If HIV could cause depression in this way, there would be a significant difference in prevalence rates of depression between HIV-positive and HIV-negative individuals. There is not.

As a diagnosis, mood disorder due to a general medical condition is more applicable to a number of indirect effects of HIV disease – including opportunistic infections, anemia, and low testosterone – when these are associated with depressed mood. These conditions exclude major depression rather than act as its cause. Although this

Table 3.   Effects of HIV Medications on Depression
and of Antidepressants on HIV

MEDICATION	USE	PSYCHOTROPIC EFFECT
EFAVIRENZ (SUSTIVA)	HIV antiviral drug	Somnolence, insomnia, vivid dreams
DRONABINOL (MARINOL)	Appetite stimulant	Apathy, somnolence
OPIATES	Pain relief	Apathy, somnolence, disorientation
TRICYCLIC ANTIDEPRESSANTS	Peripheral neuropathy relief	Partial antidepressant*

*Tricyclic antidepressants also relieve peripheral neuropathy, and in doses used to treat peripheral neuropathy, it is important to note that they may mask but not resolve depressive symptoms.

distinction may be subtle, since physical and psychological symptoms can overlap, it is crucial because the primary focus of treatment for depression due to a general medical condition should be the underlying medical condition. In assessing for a medical etiology of clinical depression, perhaps the single most important variable is the time course of the illness and the corresponding symptoms of depression. Obviously the two must be related in terms of timing. Remission of illness usually correlates with decreased depression; escalation usually correlates with increased depression.

In diagnosing a mood disorder due to medical condition, clinicians should also consider the effects of HIV-related and other medications. It is not unusual for seropositive clients to be using a variety of medications; and this is particularly true among individuals with advanced HIV disease. Several medications commonly used in the treatment of HIV can either affect depression or have been implicated as producing a symptom of depression (See Table 3: Effects of HIV Medications on Depression and of Antidepressants on HIV).

How can a clinician distinguish the physical symptoms of HIV disease from the symptoms of clinical depression? In one literature review of depression in the medically ill, the authors suggest using criteria for depression that include substitution items for these confounding symptoms.[74] First developed for use in patients with cancer, these criteria replace the somatic symptoms (the so-called vegetative signs of weight loss, sleep disturbance, fatigue, and concentration problems) with psychological ones. (See Table 4: Psychological Substitutions for HIV-Related Vegetative Symptoms for a list of these substitutions.) This approach is practical rather than academic, that is, it attempts less to distinguish a mood disorder due to a general medical condition from other forms of clinical depression; it is more concerned with differentiating clinical depression from medical illness. For the front-line clinician, this may be the most valuable distinction to make. It is important to note that vegetative symptoms remain relevant to the diagnosis of depression. Clinicians should substitute psychological indicators for physical ones only when there is reason to believe that the client's medical condition is causing physical symptoms that overlap with the vegetative symptoms used to diagnose depression.

Martha: Exacerbation by Medication

Martha, a 46-year-old, White, married woman with symptomatic HIV disease, had experienced a long history of chronic depression beginning from before her seroconversion. The depression had been under control with antidepressants and psychotherapy. Because of an increase in the viral load, Martha's primary care provider decided to change her medication regimen, including adding efavirenz. Subsequently, Martha developed an acute worsening of depressive symptoms with more frequent tearfulness and despair, profound sleep disturbance, and intense and daily suicidal ideation. These symptoms lasted a week and remitted with discontinuation of the efavirenz. Although the depressive symptoms did not completely resolve, they did return to more manageable levels, which were ultimately controlled with an increase in the sertraline dose. The presumptive diagnosis of mood disorder due to a medical condition (for the one-week exacerbation of symptoms) was able to be made because there was a tight temporal correlation between the use of efavirenz and the development of the dramatic depressive symptoms.

Table 4.   Psychological Substitutions for HIV-Related Vegetative Symptoms

Adapted with permission from: Endicott J. Measurement of depression in patients with cancer. Cancer. 1984; 53(10): 2243-2248.

VEGETATIVE SYMPTOM	PSYCHOLOGICAL SUBSTITUTION
Poor appetite or weight loss	Fearful or depressed appearance
Insomnia or hypersomnia	Social withdrawal or decreased talkativeness
Loss of energy or fatigue	Brooding affect, self-pity, or pessimism
Difficulty thinking or concentrating	Mood not reactive: cannot be cheered up; does not smile

Other Primary Depressions

In addition to major depression described above, the primary depressive disorders include bipolar depression and dysthymia. The principle distinguishing feature of bipolar depression – formerly known as manic depression – is a history of mania. Mania is characterized by an abnormally elevated or irritable mood, sleep disturbance, racing thoughts, impulsiveness, grandiosity, and extreme loquaciousness. Evaluation of a depressive disorder should always include assessing for a history of mania, since the pharmacological treatment for depression in the context of mania is mood stabilization rather than simple antidepressant regimens. It is important to note as well that there have been reports of manic syndromes induced by viral infection of the central nervous system.[75] It is not clear if this type of mania is related to accompanying depressions – as in the cyclical pattern of classic bipolar disorder or if these manic episodes stand alone.

Finally, dysthymia is a more chronic, but less severe, form of major depression, which lasts at least two years. It is possible to have concurrent dysthymia and major depression. One study found elevated rates of dysthymia among HIV-positive men with CD4+ cell counts of less than 500.[6]

Brian: Depression and Mania

Brian is a 29-year-old, Asian gay man with an AIDS diagnosis and CD4+ cell count of less than 100, who experiences classic symptoms of depression, including anhedonia and suicidality, and begins antidepressant treatment with fluoxetine. Brian's family history includes "some kind of craziness" in his maternal grandmother that had resulted in her psychiatric hospitalization. Brian responds quickly to the antidepressant, but six weeks into the treatment, he complains of irritability and interrupted sleep (only four hours each night). Brian's primary care physician adds a small amount of trazadone, another antidepressant, as a bedtime sedative. Within a week, Brian experiences a frank manic episode, sleeping only a few hours a night and talking rapidly to strangers on the street about curing HIV with an extract of oranges and bee pollen. When he presents for a follow-up medical appointment, he is demanding and extremely irritable, picking fights with other clients, while simultaneously attempting to keep a detailed catalogue of grievances on scraps of paper. He receives immediate attention by the clinic psychiatrist, who diagnoses Brian with an acute manic episode and recommends hospitalization. The mania had been precipitated by the antidepressant regimen. A more careful psychiatric history would have revealed near manic symptoms in the past.

Stress Disorders

Clinicians must consider several other psychiatric diagnoses that may present with depressed mood, although these are not, in and of themselves, full depressive disorders. One grouping of these diagnoses might be called "reactive," by which the individual responds to stressors in the external environment. Reactive diagnoses include adjustment disorders, acute stress reaction, and post-traumatic stress disorder (PTSD). The second group of diagnoses are more intrinsic and include personality disorders and other conditions related to character.

According to the DSM-IV, an adjustment disorder is the "development of emotional or behavioral symptoms in response to an identifiable stressor(s) occurring within three months of the onset of the stressor(s)." By definition, symptoms remit within six months of the termination of the stressful incident. The DSM-IV classifies adjustment disorders according to mood – depressed or anxious – and conduct – maladaptive or grossly inappropriate behaviors. In the context of HIV disease, clinicians should consider a diagnosis of adjustment disorder with depressed mood when depressive symptoms follow in the wake of a discrete "event." Unfortunately, HIV provides a great many possibilities: seroconversion, progression of illness (from asymptomatic to symptomatic, or from symptomatic to AIDS), change in markers of progression (such as CD4+ cell counts or viral load readings), and failure of medication regimens. The depressive symptoms associated with an adjustment disorder are marked and cause a loss of normal function, but they do not have the severity of a major depressive disorder. Meeting the criteria for major depression automatically excludes a diagnosis of adjustment disorder with depressed mood.

Similarly, acute stress disorder and post-traumatic stress disorder may lead to depressive symptoms in response to specific occurrences. At the heart of both types of stress disorder diagnoses is a traumatic event that involves "actual or threatened death or serious injury." The difference between acute and post-traumatic stress disorders is largely a temporal one: acute stress is more circumscribed, occurring within the month of the traumatic event; post-traumatic stress lasts more than a month. In both cases, the individual responds to this event by reexperiencing it through dreams, flashbacks, or intrusive recollections, or by distancing it through numbing, dissociation, or avoidance. While the basic mood is one of anxiety and hyperarousal rather than depression, avoidance and dissociation can be mistaken for the anhedonia of depression. Many HIV-positive individuals have had harrowing experiences, witnessing the illness, decline, and death of partner and friends. Some have literally lost their entire network of social support. Additionally, childhood sexual trauma may predispose some individuals to high-risk behaviors that ultimately result in their HIV infection. In individuals with PTSD, recurrent loss, complicated bereavement, or traumatic memories, HIV disease represents a new trauma often leading to symptoms of sadness, depressed numbness, and anxiety. In fact, individuals suffering from stress disorders often develop a superimposed, full-blown, clinical depression.

Manuel: Acute Stress Disorder

Manuel is a 35-year-old, heterosexual, Mexican man who has lived in the United States for two months. He is undocumented and speaks only a little English. His wife and two children remain in their small hometown in northern Mexico, living with Manuel's parents. Because of physical symptoms, including a chronic cough and malaise, Manuel was screened for tuberculosis and later for HIV as part of a health program for day laborers. The results indicated that he was HIV-infected. He was referred to a city clinic, where his doctor started him on an HIV antiviral regimen.

Manuel debated whether to tell his family – particularly since he was ashamed that he might have become infected through sex with prostitutes – but he finally wrote his wife with the news. When he called his home two weeks later, his mother informed him that his wife had left with the two children, saying she no longer wanted to see Manuel. Manuel's impulse was to return to Mexico, but social workers at the clinic advised him against it because he would probably have difficulty obtaining antiviral medications. Manuel came in for a mental health evaluation with the following symptoms: daily anxiety attacks, poor concentration, tearfulness, insomnia, a sense that he was "not himself," and recurrent thoughts of suicide. Although Manuel displayed prominent depressive symptoms, he was also given a diagnosis of acute stress disorder, because his anxiety symptoms seemed to be in response to the traumatic events he had recently experienced.

Personality Disorders

Personality disorders are characterized by patterns of thinking, emotional expression, interpersonal function, and impulse control that significantly impair social functioning. Individuals with personality disorders often have problematic relationships, including with their providers. A relatively simple negotiation about treatment can turn into a volatile power struggle, and establishing a human connection with the client can seem a Herculean task. Clinical depression in clients with personality disorders is diagnosable using the standard DSM-IV criteria, that is, personality disorders and clinical depressions (such as major depressive episode or dysthymia) are separate, but sometimes coincident, entities. Often clients with personality disorders do not respond as robustly to antidepressant treatment as those without a concurrent personality disorder. It is as if the depression itself becomes a part of the personality of the individual, and its removal threatens structural damage.

Frederick: Personality Disorder and Dysthymia

Frederick is a 40-year-old, single, gay man with a history of marginal employment who now has disabling AIDS and lives in a residential setting that provides social support services. His presenting mental health complaints include irritability, depressed mood, frequent tearfulness, low self-esteem, and a sense that "no one respects me." A disagreement with a housemate over the use of the kitchen escalated into a violent verbal confrontation. Frederick superficially cut his left wrist in his room afterwards, and was then taken to the emergency room. At his follow-up appointment with a clinic psychiatrist, Frederick told his psychiatrist about his earlier suicide attempts and psychiatric hospitalizations, leading to the conclusion that he met criteria for dysthymia and a non-specific personality disorder.

After a careful and thorough evaluation, Frederick's psychiatrist interpreted the suicide attempt as an expression of anger, rather than as a desire to die. The superficiality of the cuts and their quick public display by Frederick provided some reassurance that his actual risk of suicide was low. Frederick explained that he "almost always" thought of suicide and had been doing so since his teenage years when he had left his abusive childhood home. The suicidal thoughts had worsened since he was diagnosed with AIDS a year previously. About his depression and low self-esteem he stated: "They have been with me as long as I can remember." Frederick started taking an antidepressant and began psychotherapy. A year later, he was less frequently tearful, but still became easily irritated with others. Increasingly, however, this irritation was directed at his therapist, rather than at his housemates, and he expressed his feelings rather than acting them out in suicide attempts.

Character and Resiliency

While depression is a clinical entity, the person suffering from it is not. The diagnosis of depression should always be placed in the context of an individual's life narrative and cultural surround. Every individual has strengths of character and sources of resiliency. Part of the depression assessment should be to discover and highlight these areas, to observe whether a buoyant sense of humor or a dogged survival stubbornness mitigates the effects of depression.[76] Such an affirmation can help establish a strong alliance between client and clinician, forming the foundation of other treatment interventions. It can also become the basis of a preventative strategy against the threat of future episodes of depression, suggesting how to build on the strengths of the client and balance liabilities.

HIV disease, after all, often represents a recurrently traumatizing situation as disease progresses, and managing treatment and progression requires psychological stamina. Many individuals manage this stress without developing psychiatric dysfunction. Those who do develop clinically significant depression may have a combination of predispositions. Some will have an inherited tendency to depression or a biological vulnerability due to an insult to the central nervous system. Others may feel overwhelmed and alone because they do not have the social support necessary to help them cope with the stress of the illness. This may be the result of multiple losses dissipating support networks, of cultural barriers that isolate individuals by stigmatizing them, or of self-imposed prohibitions that cut individuals off from others. Biological predisposition, psychological resiliency, and social support may balance each other out, with strength in one area making up for deficits in another. When external stressors such as HIV disease, tip this balance, the result is clinical depression.

Conclusion

Whether HIV independently promotes depression in those who are HIV-infected remains unclear. Despite methodological constraints, however, epidemiological data do seem to point unequivocally to two things: clinically significant depression is not uncommon in individuals who are HIV-infected; and for many subgroups, stigmatizing social factors, such as being gay or an injection drug user, may be more significant than HIV infection itself in causing depression. Being HIV-positive may further this process of stigmatization.

The interactions between social context and internal psychology, between the biological substrate of the brain and the virtual structure of the mind, are complex and incompletely understood. But, it seems reasonable to postulate a model that attempts to understand the function of HIV disease as an entity that can operate at all of these levels simultaneously. As a virus, HIV leaves the body vulnerable to illness and malaise, factors that may erode resilience. As a psychological insult that threatens integrity and induces uncertainty, the idea of HIV exposes the self to enormous stress. And as a social force, the stigma of HIV disrupts and reconfigures social networks, at times making cultural outsiders of those whom it labels. Clinicians need to consider all of this complexity as they assess clients with depressive symptoms in order to ensure the most appropriate treatment.

4

Interventions and Treatments

Two principles form the foundation of treatment for HIV-related depression. First, since HIV affects the individual simultaneously in physical, psychological, and social ways, it is crucial to operate on these three levels, and ideal to establish a collaboration among a team of providers that can adequately address these multiple concerns in a coordinated fashion. Second, since depression is essentially a response to loss, it is essential to foster a strong therapeutic alliance, one that emphasizes the protective environment of a trusting relationship. Adhering to these principles, treatment modalities fall into two groups: pharmacological and psychotherapeutic. This chapter focuses on the development of a treatment plan that integrates these modalities.

Working within a Multidisciplinary Team

Because of the complexities of issues involved in working with HIV, the multidisciplinary team has emerged as a common mechanism for the delivery of care. Composed of medical providers, social workers, mental health personnel, and other providers (including nutritionists, treatment advocates, legal and financial counselors, and peer support staff), the team is better equipped than unaffiliated providers to manage HIV in a coordinated and effective manner. Some groups of providers, housed in one clinic or agency, work together explicitly as a team; but more often, providers from different agencies or offices form a "virtual" team and improvise a way to coordinate care. In both cases, communication can be a challenge, and when it collapses, the results can be deleterious for treatment.

Communication between mental health and primary care providers is mutually beneficial to the goals of both teams. Drug interactions between psychotropic medications and some HIV medications, for example, are dangerous and relatively common, so when antidepressants are prescribed, it is important for a client's psychiatrist and primary care physician to maintain current medication lists. Likewise, adherence to complicated HIV regimens can be extremely difficult, and primary care physicians would be wise to consider psychiatric treatment or social work interventions as a fundamental part of the HIV medical treatment plan. Finally, communication between a non-psychiatrist psychotherapist and a consulting psychiatrist ensures coordination of interventions and provides a framework for making treatment decisions. At times a client will need to recognize, experience, and integrate depressive affects in order to get better and this may suggest an emphasis on psychotherapy; at other times, these affective states need to be recognized as products of depressive illness, and this may require prioritizing pharmacological intervention.

When several providers are involved, as is often the case with HIV-related care, there is a greater likelihood of "splitting." Splitting is a psychotherapeutic concept, which for the purposes of this discussion refers to a fragmentation of care into discrete entities. Clients will sometimes project their own ambivalence about psychological conflicts onto various team members, telling different providers different parts of the their story. For example, a client may tell one provider about his or her drug use, but not mention it to another. Usually, splitting is not a deliberate manipulation by the client, and providers should instead interpret it as a sign of inadequate coordination on the part of the team. Splitting can be a particularly vexing issue when there is more than one prescribing physician, for example when there is a primary care physician and a psychiatrist, resulting in muddled polypharmacology.

When splitting is the problem or when there is disagreement among providers about treatment goals, a case conference can help to establish therapeutic priorities. For instance, in the case of a client whose depression manifests as a passive wish to die but who is a prime candidate for an aggressive antiviral regimen, providers might well agree to stabilize the depression first, rather than run the risk of poor adherence to antiviral treatment and the development of viral resistance. In a client with substance abuse issues and depression, a case conference can turn a shameful secret into a resolvable problem, in which all members of the health care team can take a supportive role.

The Therapeutic Relationship

The establishment of a strong therapeutic alliance between provider and client is clearly the fundamental goal of any treatment approach, whether medical or psychological. Because of the extreme social stigma that is still attached to HIV, many seropositive individuals harbor buried feelings of guilt and shame. In psychotherapy, these emotions often surface only after therapist and client have undertaken considerable work to establish a sense of security in the therapeutic relationship. Additionally, HIV represents a major life trauma or rupture, dividing life into "before HIV" and "after HIV." It promotes an identity shift, as individuals struggle to integrate a life-threatening illness into their sense of who they are and what the future holds. Further, HIV changes the quality of a person's relationships, often leading to secrecy and creating an instant "closet." It can require wrenching decisions, as seropositive individuals decide to whom to disclose and face the possibility of isolation and discrimination.

The psychotherapeutic relationship, founded on confidence and trust, provides a haven in which these conflicts and traumas can be faced. But to some extent, all relationships with HIV providers serve this function and probably help to alleviate pressures of social stigma and anxieties about the physical and psychological insults of HIV. Empathetic and caring providers may well provide some protection against depression, one etiology of which is the lack of social support.

The significance of the provider-client relationship as a therapeutic factor should not be overlooked by medical practitioners, who obviously do much more than manage illness and medications. For many patients, the medical practitioner represents protection, a sense of control, and hope. It is common to hear from individuals who have felt anxious when they did not have easy access to their primary care providers or despondent when there were conflicts in these medical relationships. Conversely, for patients for whom it is clear that their doctor is "on their side," the medical relationship instills psychological strength and encouragement.

The medical provider is among the most powerful allies the patient can have in the battle with HIV. Fears that this provider does not really want to help the patient, worries about his or her competence, and concerns about real or psychological availability can seriously shake the patient's sense of being supported. Differences in the quality of provider-patient relationships are not exclusively the function of the patient's ability to access the physician's medical care; they are also a result of a provider's dexterity in recognizing and responding to the psychological aspects of the medical relationship, a relationship, that while not *psychotherapy,* has the potential of being *psychotherapeutic.*

Medical and Pharmacological Interventions

Antidepressant medications provide a powerful and effective remedy for most types of clinical depression and constitute the mainstay of treatment and standard of care for major depression. In response to other depressive syndromes – such as adjustment disorders with depressed mood, grief and complicated bereavement, substance-induced depressive disorders, characterologically based depressions, and even dysthymia – clinicians have differing thresholds for recommending psychopharmacological evaluation. Because contemporary antidepressants are safe and have relatively few side effects, providers often prescribe trials of antidepressant medication for even relatively mild depression. The greatest danger of antidepressants is that some clients may overmedicalize symptoms, that is, develop the expectation that medication is the only remedy for their ills, preventing them from developing the necessary psychological skills for better functioning.

As emphasized earlier, treatment for depression is most effective when coordinated using a team approach. The prescription of psychotropic medication is no exception. Antidepressants should be seen as one tool for coping, rather than as the cure for depression: antidepressants provide a "floor" to keep clients from sinking, enabling them to "stand up" so they can better handle the hard work of psychotherapy or HIV disease management. In some cases, for example, significant cognitive impairment, traditional psychotherapy may not be appropriate or a client may simply refuse therapy; but even in these cases, the therapeutic value of relationships with medical providers, case managers, or other providers often play a critical role in treatment.

To understand the role of antidepressant medications, it is useful to review the etiology of depression. Biological and genetic predispositions establish the basic risk for becoming depressed in response to trauma; psychological and social factors provide extra liability or protection given the particular circumstances. Thus, a client whose mother suffered severe clinical depressions requiring hospitalization may be at risk on two fronts: a genetic predisposition and a psychological predisposition resulting from a relatively unavailable mother. This client may be fortified by a close network of friends or further hampered by being relatively isolated. When struck by an HIV-related traumatic event, this client may be prone to developing clinical depression. Antidepressant treatment would be a logical intervention (particularly given his or her family history), but even a good response to medication does not obviate psychotherapy. While emotions are probably ultimately mediated by biological mechanisms, all depression has subjective meanings for the individual experiencing it. Thus, a fundamental premise of this monograph is that multiple levels of intervention are critical.

In most simple cases of first-time depression, antidepressants should be a time-limited intervention, used strategically and based on clear target symptoms. Six months after a full remission of depressive symptoms – in the case of a simple major depressive episode – the provider should attempt to wean the client from medications. It is often useful for the client to continue in psychotherapy for some time after the discontinuation of antidepressants to ensure there is no relapse. Clients with recurrent depressions, on the other hand, require longer treatment periods, lasting at least a year, and may even need to take medication for life depending on age and the number and severity of previous episodes. Cases should be managed on an individual basis, with a careful analysis of the risks and benefits of continuing or discontinuing antidepressant treatment.

Most primary, non-psychiatrist, medical providers are comfortable managing medications for uncomplicated depressions such as dysthymia or an initial and mild to moderate major depressive episode. When starting antidepressant treatment, medical providers should consider whether patients might benefit from psychotherapy. In cases where the patient does begin psychotherapy, the medical provider should be available to the therapist for consultation and coordination of medication treatment and to avoid splitting. Ideally, the therapist and medical provider will confer: the medical provider should alert the therapist to dose or medication changes; conversely, the therapist can help monitor side effects and treatment efficacy. For more complicated depressions, such as recurrent major depression (especially when resistant to treatment), acutely suicidal depressions of any type, any depression requiring psychiatric hospitalization, or bipolar or psychotic depressions, most primary care providers should refer clients to a psychiatrist. Primary medical providers should also consider referring depressed patients with personality disorders, who require a consistent clinical approach and may require a great deal of attention.

In most cases, the presence of HIV does not change the basic principles for prescribing antidepressant medications, particularly in asymptomatic or mildly symptomatic HIV-positive clients. As with uninfected individuals, the choice of an antidepressant is based on efficacy of past treatments, a family history of good response to an agent, the side effect profile of the agent, and the ancillary benefit of side effects to the client. Many HIV-positive patients are already taking an impressive list of drugs, sometimes exceeding twenty pills a day. The complexities of these regimens, with multiple dosings each day and different requirements regarding meals, has been widely recognized. In addition, these medications all have side effects, ranging from diarrhea and nausea to headaches and malaise to sleeplessness. The addition of another drug – an antidepressant – with more potential side effects and interactions, should be undertaken with care. It is advisable to "start low and go slow" in dosing psychotropic medication, especially if a client is already taking a variety of medications or has advanced HIV disease. Given these caveats, however, the clinician should not hold back from treating seropositive clients with pharmacological interventions. Whenever possible, side effects should be matched to the particular individual in such a way that they become ancillary benefits rather than handicaps: for example, a sedating antidepressant for the person with insomnia, and a stimulating one for the individual with lethargy.

HIV antiviral drugs can have potentially dangerous interactions with some psychoactive compounds. The interactions occur primarily because HIV drugs can inhibit the activity of liver enzymes, which are responsible for the metabolization and degradation of various chemical substances, including medications. (See Table 5: Potential Interactions between HIV Antiviral Drugs and Psychotropic Medications.) As a result, HIV treatments can radically increase the effective amount of a drug in circulation, sometimes to toxic levels. While identifying drug interactions has become increasingly complex as scientists discover more and more about the specific pharmacodynamics of many medications, the general provider should be aware, at least, of the interactions with ritonavir (Norvir). This protease inhibitor can interfere with the metabolism of a number of psychoactive medicines, including many benzodiazepines (such as temazepam) and some antidepressants. Buproprion (Wellbutrin) is theoretically contraindicated with ritonavir, but in clinical practice, the two are sometimes used together with careful monitoring.

The Antidepressants

There is a wide range of antidepressant agents – easily more than twenty commonly used medications. They have varying mechanisms of action and pharmacodynamics. Chief among these are the selective serotonin reuptake inhibitors (SSRI), the tricyclic antidepressants, and the atypical agents.

Most psychiatrists today use an SSRI as the first line in the treatment of most problematic depressive symptoms. The SSRIs have the advantage of being relatively well-tolerated, safe, and having few interactions with other types of medication. In the context of HIV, some of the more difficult secondary effects of the SSRIs are gastrointestinal, including nausea and anorexia. Anorexia can be especially troubling in individuals who already suffer from weight loss or wasting. However, appetite sometimes improves after initiation of SSRI treatment, since loss of appetite is also a symptom of depression. It is important to note that many side effects improve after a week or two of treatment as the body accommodates the medication.

The side effect that most often leads to discontinuation of SSRI treatment is sexual dysfunction. Sexual dysfunction occurs frequently, most usually causing a marked decrease in sexual interest (libido), poor sexual function (diminished erections or vaginal lubrication or pain on insertion), or changes in the quality or rapidity of orgasm. Time to orgasm is usually delayed, with anorgasmia (inability to have an orgasm) resulting in the more extreme cases. The subjective response to these effects are varied. The typical response is frustration

Table 5. Potential Interactions between HIV Antiviral Drugs and Psychotropic Medications

HIV antiviral drugs are most likely to interact with the sedative/hypnotics (antianxiety and sleep medications) and with anticonvulsant agents, both of which are sometimes used to treat complicated depressions. This table provides a sample of some of these interactions, some of which are theoretical rather than clinically established. When in doubt about a possible interaction, consult with a knowledgeable pharmacist.

ANTIVIRAL	PSYCHOTROPIC	EFFECT
Protease Inhibitors (PIs)		
Amprenavir (Agenerase) Indinavir (Crixivan) Nelfinavir (Viracept) Saquinivir (Invirase)	Carbamazepine (Tegretol)	Decrease in HIV antiviral drug level
	Diazepam (Valium) Flurazepam (Dalmane) Triazolam (Halcion)	Increase in psychotropic drug level; potential toxicity
Ritonavir (Norvir)	Amitriptyline (Elavil) Buproprion (Wellbutrin) Desipramine (Norpramin) Diazepam (Valium) Fluoxetine (Prozac) Flurazepam (Dalmane) Nefazadone (Serzone) Sertraline (Zoloft) Triazolam (Halcion) Zoldipem (Ambien)	Increase in psychotropic drug level; potential toxicity
Non-Nucleoside Reverse Transcriptase Inhibitors (NNRTIs)		
Delavirdine (Rescriptor) Efavirenz (Sustiva) Nevirapine (Viramune)	Carbamazepine (Tegretol)	Decrease in HIV antiviral drug level
Delavirdine (Rescriptor)	Fluoxetine (Prozac)	Increase in HIV antiviral drug level
	Diazepam (Valium) Flurazepam (Dalmane) Triazolam (Halcion)	Increase in psychotropic drug level; potential toxicity

and discontent, but some individuals such as men who have a history of premature ejaculation may welcome some of these side effects as salutary. Management of sexual dysfunction includes dose reduction, carefully orchestrated medication holidays (in which the client temporarily discontinues the antidepressant regimen), and the addition of a number of questionable agents to enhance sexual performance. More often, the solution is to switch to an agent without these problems, for example, buproprion (Wellbutrin) or nefazadone (Serzone). Based on anecdotal evidence, low doses of buproprion can also be added to the SSRIs to help counteract sexual dysfunction.

A number of studies have demonstrated the efficacy of the SSRIs in the treatment of depression for HIV-positive individuals.[77] Among the various agents to choose from, fluoxetine (Prozac) tends to be more stimulating, while paroxetine (Paxil) is more sedating. A newer SSRI, citalopram (Celexa), seems to have few drug interactions.

Since they are more easily tolerated and safer, the SSRIs displaced the equally effective tricyclic antidepressants as the standard treatment for depression in the 1980s. Tricyclic antidepressants have a strong affinity for anticholinergic receptors in the brain, which can result in a host of side effects: dry mouth, constipation, urinary retention, and blurred vision. They also tend to be sedating. There have been reports of significantly higher discontinuation rates among HIV-positive clients taking tricyclic antidepressants when compared to sedating SSRIs.[78] This is probably due to the greater frequency of other bothersome effects. One of the most dangerous aspects of these medications is that, unlike SSRIs, they are lethal in overdose (a fatal dose is usually about one gram), contraindicating them in acutely suicidal individuals.

Tricyclic antidepressants (TCAs) can be useful for clients with peripheral neuropathy – especially in the context of insomnia – since these drugs may alleviate neuropathic pain while simultaneously helping with sleep. At times, they can be judiciously combined with SSRIs for treatment-resistant depressions or for peripheral neuropathy, but this should be undertaken cautiously, since SSRIs increase tricyclic antidepressant levels. Since tricyclic antidepressants in high doses can cause irregular heart rhythms, they should not be used in clients with HIV-related heart conditions (such as cardiomyopathy).

Atypical antidepressants include buproprion (Wellbutrin) and mirtazapine (Remeron). Buproprion has emerged as a useful agent because it is virtually free of sexual side effects, and so can be an alternative to the SSRIs. Generally well-tolerated, buproprion's greatest disadvantage is that it apparently lowers the seizure threshold at doses of more than 450 milligrams per day (although some reports have found that the incidence of seizure activity at this dose is comparable to other antidepressants).[79] As mentioned above, the protease inhibitor ritonavir theoretically causes a marked increase in buproprion levels. Mirtazapine is a sedating atypical antidepressant that typically causes an increase in appetite. This side effect, often a significant impediment in general practice, can be a boon in seropositive individuals with wasting syndrome.

In prescribing antidepressants, medical providers should keep in mind cultural factors. In one study of 118 depressed HIV-positive patients treated with fluoxetine for eight weeks, researchers found greater attrition by Latinos than either Whites or Blacks. Latinos were also more likely to respond to placebo than participants from the other two groups, whereas Blacks were less likely to respond to fluoxetine than Whites. There was no difference among the groups in terms of side effects.[80] While this is a single, and perhaps idiosyncratic, study, it points to potential differences in medications based on ethnicity. Sociocultural factors, including spiritual beliefs and the perceived power and beneficence of the provider, might affect adherence to regimens and psychological effects (such as the placebo effect).

Other Medications

It is important for providers to be aware of a number of other medications used to treat depressive disorders. Among these are sedatives and sleep aids, mood stabilizers, psychostimulants, and testosterone.

Sedatives and Sleep Aids

Insomnia is one of the most common complaints of HIV-positive clients with depression. As noted earlier, as many as 73 percent of people with HIV suffer from insomnia, which can be caused by a variety of factors. As a cardinal symptom of clinical depression, insomnia will usually resolve with antidepressant treatment. In these cases it can be helpful to employ a sedating antidepressant such as one of the tricyclics, paroxetine, nefazadone, or mirtazapine.

When additional medications are necessary, benzodiazepines – for example, triazolam (Halcion), temazepam (Restoril), and lorazepam (Ativan) – are among the most common hypnotics. These medications are useful over courses of one to two weeks, but over longer periods, they can increase both cognitive deficits and depression, cause dependence, and diminish sexual function. As mentioned earlier, some protease inhibitors, notably ritonavir, can significantly increase the plasma concentration of many of the benzodiazepines with the potentially dangerous consequences of oversedation or coma. Trazadone (Desyrel), an atypical antidepressant, rarely used any longer because of its severely sedating effects at therapeutic doses, is very useful in low doses to treat insomnia. It does not cause dependence, but it sometimes produces a "hangover" effect and dizziness. Zoldipem (Ambien), which binds selective benzodiazepine receptors, can also be useful, although it can lead to dependence. As with any sleep medication that can cause dependence, it should only be used for short periods (about two weeks).

The treatment of insomnia should not be seen as the exclusive purview of pharmacology. Instead, clinicians should take a careful sleep history and recommend behavioral interventions. These include the development of good sleep hygiene (regular sleep/wake schedules, daily exercise, minimal intake of caffeine, nicotine, drugs and alcohol, and avoidance of naps). Clients can help regularize their sleep/wake schedules by going to bed at approximately the same time every night and using an alarm clock in the morning. When clients have difficulty falling asleep, they should not remain sleepless in bed for more than twenty to thirty minutes, since this practice can habituate the mind to use the bed as a place of worry and rumination. Rather, clients should get up and do something calming, for example, have a snack or warm milk, sit in a rocking chair, or read, and wait until they become sleepy again. Behavioral interventions can take more of a clinician's time, since they require working on habits that are often ingrained, and regular monitoring. But behavioral approaches are at least as effective as pharmacological interventions, and for the clients who are already taking a number of HIV-related medications, they eliminate risky drug interactions and additional side effects.

Mood Stabilizers

Treating depression in the context of bipolar disorder requires a mood stabilizer, since use of only an antidepressant may promote manic episodes. Mood stabilizers have antidepressant effect, but when this is insufficient to control depression, it may be necessary to add an antidepressant drug. Lithium, the gold standard for the treatment of classic bipolar disorder, is often not the best agent to use in the context of HIV disease. Lithium is a salt, and as such is exquisitely sensitive to "volume status," the water balance in a person's body. More importantly, lithium has a very narrow therapeutic window, and so can become toxic with relatively small changes in the dose. HIV and the antiviral medications used to treat it can disrupt volume status, mostly through diarrhea and other gastrointestinal disturbances. A sudden loss of total body water can increase the concentration of lithium precipitously, leading to toxicity and loss of coordination, seizures, cerebellar damage, and even coma. The newer anticonvulsant mood stabilizers, including valproate (Depakote), lamotrigine (Lamictal), and gabapentin (Neurontin), can be used with HIV-related medications. The atypical antipsychotic olanzapine (Zyprexa) has also recently been approved for treatment of acute mania. Most mood stabilizers can cause drowsiness or fatigue, which usually resolves over the first few weeks of use.

Psychostimulants

The psychostimulants, including dextroamphetamine (Biphetamine), methylphenidate (Ritalin), and pemoline (Cylert), are sometimes used in the treatment of depression in the medically ill because they have a rapid onset of action, few adverse effects, and minimal drug interactions. They are, however, highly controlled substances, and this limits their wide use. They require triplicate prescriptions, obtainable from the Drug Enforcement Administration (DEA), and cannot be authorized for refills. They also have "street value," restricting their use in some patients with significant drug abuse issues. Finally, there is the association, in the minds of both provider and client, between psychostimulants and illicit substances, which might have a psychologically inhibiting effect. Psychostimulants are sometimes used to treat HIV-related dementia, notably without abuse or dependence,[81] and seem to be the logical choice to treat depression in the context of cognitive impairment. They are also being studied for treatment of HIV-related fatigue.[82]

Testosterone

Typically, testosterone is used in HIV-related care to respond to wasting syndrome in individuals with symptoms of hypogonadism, which include low libido, low mood, low energy, and loss of appetite and weight. In a trial to evaluate testosterone therapy, 79 percent of

HIV-positive men with major depressive disorder or dysthymia reported significant improvement of mood after eight weeks of treatment.[83] Both men with and without testosterone deficiency showed response to treatment for hypogonadic symptoms. Treatment was well-tolerated.

Psychological and Psychotherapeutic Interventions

While uncomplicated cases of mild to moderate clinical depression may be effectively managed with antidepressant medication and supportive listening by the primary care provider, some individuals need much more. Since clinical depressions can be conceptualized as the failure of a personal "system" that includes a psychological subject in the context of his or her sociocultural surroundings, psychotherapy is critical to comprehensive treatment. In most cases, if an individual is depressed enough to benefit from antidepressants, he or she will probably benefit from psychotherapy; and many clients will benefit from therapy long before they develop the clinical symptoms that require antidepressant intervention. At a minimum, medical providers should consider referring for psychotherapy those clinically depressed patients who are suicidal, particularly those with a history of suicide attempts, who have significant problems in managing relationships, who have a history of trauma, or who have experienced acute loss or chronic multiple losses. Psychotherapy may also be a useful adjunct in the management of HIV medication adherence when adherence issues are a manifestation of internal conflicts or self-destructive impulses.

Psychotherapy offers clients a protected professional relationship in which to rework psychological templates or to change entrenched and obsolete ways of thinking. Using a computer analogy, if medications help alter the hard-wiring of the brain, psychotherapy retools the software. Medication support and psychotherapy usually work most effectively when used conjointly. Clinical depression promotes rigidity and defeatism. Antidepressants can help relieve this entrenchment – fostering the flexibility and resilience necessary to experience painful emotions – allowing an opportunity for alternatives to emerge. Psychotherapy is the process of imagining these alternatives and working to put them into action. A comprehensive description of how this kind of work gets accomplished in therapy is beyond the limits of this monograph.

Psychotherapy today encompasses a wide variety of techniques, theoretical orientations, and time courses. Which modalities are the most helpful for individuals with depression and HIV? As noted below, the research literature does favor some theoretical approaches over others, but since HIV-positive individuals present with complex circumstances and differing kinds of depressive symptoms, psychotherapeutic treatments must be tailored to the individual. This requires an array of technical approaches, some of which will be discussed below.

It should be noted that the relationship between HIV and depression is in many ways arbitrary: no person's depression can be characterized only in the context of HIV. Yoking HIV and depression together in psychotherapy can be artificial and even unproductive. A person is obviously much more than his or her HIV status, and while HIV-related concerns may initiate psychotherapeutic engagement, they should not constrict it. HIV-related issues may at times function as a defense, a kind of smoke screen that can obscure more fundamental issues such as pernicious substance abuse. Often the psychological problems highlighted by HIV are the tip of an iceberg, representing, for example, an underlying trauma. Having said this, HIV is often a powerful frame for psychotherapy. Among the key issues all therapists working with HIV and depression should consider are:

- The conflict between supporting and confronting denial;
- The unfolding of disease progression and milestones;
- The effects of these conditions on clients' cognitive abilities;
- The shape of the psychotherapeutic frame;
- The relationship between past trauma and HIV.

To Confront or Support Denial?

One of the most fundamental dynamics with which all therapists work is the balance between sustaining useful adaptive denial and confronting painful realities. HIV-related therapy brings this tension into relief. The meanings of HIV are as varied as each individual. Even in the age of combination antiviral treatment, for many, HIV still represents mortality, the enactment of a hidden self-destructive urge, the shameful badge of an outcast, or the price of desire. Some of these meanings are clear and on the surface of the client's consciousness; others slowly emerge during the course of therapy or may seem evident to the therapist and not to the client.

Therapists working with HIV routinely face the dilemma of deciding when to suggest tackling a protective defense against a painful truth versus supporting the defense in the service of "happier existence." Over-interpreting a client's defenses can leave him or her uselessly and painfully exposed or even compromise functioning; after all, denial is an essential part of living, allowing selective attention to a given task. On the other hand, denial can be insidious and destructive: consider the virulent denial of the alcoholic, or of the individual who, disavowing all risk, seroconverts. One guideline therapists can use in determining whether to confront denial is the level of a client's current and future functioning. When denial about the harsh realities of HIV sustains the client's ability to live fully, for example, by minimizing the inconvenience of minor side effects, a therapist might silently support this avoidance of difficulty. But when denial interferes with a client's ability to care for him or herself, a therapist should consider empathic confrontation. In some cases, this includes confronting the denial of death in order to help a dying client deal with unfinished business.

Disease Progression and Milestones

HIV disease represents a series of thresholds for clients: from seroconversion to the development of symptoms to increasing illness and possible incapacitation to terminal illness. At these nodal points, clients are vulnerable to trauma, crises, stress reactions, and adjustment disorders. The major tasks of the therapist in responding to this evolution are to facilitate the client's stability and to help the client integrate knowledge. Usually, the approach is more supportive than explorative, with a major focus on containing and tolerating intense affect and on maintaining a realistic focus that includes hope and the possibility of control or action. Therapists need to be vigilant of the rise of depressive feelings at key points. As part of the integration of a traumatic reality, sadness and loss are normal reactions. Avoidance of such emotions may in fact promote clinical depression. Therapists should seek to help clients feel without becoming overwhelmed by their emotions.

In advanced disease, sessions are often focused on existential concerns. Clients may review broad themes in their lives, in an attempt to come to peace with their triumphs and disappointments, or they may focus on particularly agonizing treatment decisions, unresolved conflicts in close relationships, or their loss of independence and control.

The Cognitive Abilities of the Client

Therapists working with HIV-positive individuals must be mindful of the impact of organic cognitive impairment on clients with depression. As mentioned in Chapter Three, symptoms of depression and dementia can mimic one another, and depression can present with dementia or milder cognitive impairments. In such situations, the therapist must work with depression in a context of impairments that limit the client's ability to process information and emotions.

In the most straightforward cases of depression and dementia, a client's depressive feelings stem from the limitations brought about by cognitive problems. For example, a client may feel an acute sense of loss, disorientation, and anxiety after realizing that he or she is less able to manage personal affairs because of forgetfulness and poor concentration. In such cases, the therapist must alter the frame and technique of the treatment, moving away from psychodynamic and exploratory approaches toward more concrete and practical interventions.[84] For instance, a therapeutic approach that emphasizes the use of calendars and other reminder aids and encourages a greater reliance on others for the management of daily activities can help improve a client's sense of independence and minimize helplessness. Ironically, in advanced cases of dementing processes, clients often exhibit "la belle indifférence," a profound nonchalance about even dramatic impairment that is, itself, a byproduct of cognitive breakdown.

In more difficult cases, dementia and depression overlap in complicated ways. A client may suffer from a previously existing depression and develop an overlay of cognitive impairment, which only exacerbates frustration, anxiety, and agitation as the client loses the capacity to fully understand what is occurring emotionally. This is sometimes the case for the client with end-stage AIDS, who may be struggling with unresolved conflicts and other existential issues related to dying. In some cases, the failure of memory eases the tension, as the client simply "forgets" about these conflicts. Or the combination of dementia and depression may sink the client into quiet withdrawal and profound isolation. But in other cases, the client finds him or herself overwhelmed and disoriented and responds with frustration, anger, and even violence. These depressive states are usually agitated, characterized by anxiety and irritability. Such clients can be very demanding and profoundly taxing to caregivers.

In response, therapists must perform a balancing act of interventions, both providing the structuring and behavioral work required to manage the dementia and processing broader issues related to the depression. Often, widening the therapeutic frame to include family members or friends can be helpful. In these cases, the therapist can provide education that can help caregivers to reframe their expectations and to be less reactive to the client's emotions and more attentive to the client's needs. Therapists working this way may need to be more directive with clients and their loved ones, recognizing that clarity and direction can help to contain the anxiety, and thereby facilitate a process by which a family can cope together.

The Shape of the Psychotherapeutic Frame

The trauma imposed by HIV infection strongly influences the frame of psychotherapy. Therapists must sometimes modify their techniques and be more flexible about scheduling, length of sessions, place of meetings, and kinds of interventions, particularly to accommodate clients who are seriously ill. In treating people with end-stage disease, it may be more important for the therapist to be accessible than analytical, for example, meeting a client at home or holding a client's hand. In such cases, therapists may also be more willing to disclose personal information.

Depression almost always takes on some sort of somatic expression, including fatigue, pain, a dull "heartache," or a restricted affect. Many approaches to therapy treat these bodily manifestations of depression as metaphors. Within the context of HIV, this issue becomes more complicated, since HIV itself can cause a variety of physical ailments. Additionally, in cultures that make less of a distinction between mind and body (such as traditional Latino and Asian cultures), somatic concerns may also be common symptoms of depression. In response, therapists can neither react to every somatic manifestation nor merely interpret away these symptoms; they must both acknowledge the physical and work with the psychological aspects of it. First, therapists should advocate medical evaluation of physical symptoms and empower clients to make their medical needs known; likewise, they should attempt to understand and interpret any reluctance on a client's part to seek out such evaluation. Second, many clients need time to "vent" about their aches and pains, and empathic listening sends the message that the therapist is able to tolerate the discomfort and tedium of physical distress. Finally, therapists should use these opportunities to better understand how clients manage physical distress (for example, are clients seeking medical help?), to interpret the psychological significance of somatic events (is focusing on the body a way for clients to avoid feelings of sadness?), and to help clients develop methods for coping with pain (do clients know how to use relaxation or distraction?).

Questions about the psychotherapeutic frame may also arise in the context of the relationship between the therapist and the medical treatment team. For example, non-adherence to HIV antiviral regimens is one manifestation of depression; to what extent might the therapist and the medical team collaborate on promoting adherence? Therapists face an ethical danger in this situation, potentially usurping the client's agency as the ultimate arbiter of medical decisions. But, therapists can mitigate such complications by making their conflicts explicit to clients and remaining focused on client-centered goals.

Finally, the frame of HIV-related therapy is affected by time limitations: the end of the hour, the duration of treatment, and termination of therapy. As a signifier of mortality, HIV can accentuate any question of "ending," and time limitations can increase the anxiety of some clients. But the sense of limitation can also impel and catalyze the treatment. Some writers have even suggested that time limitations improve the prognosis of brief treatments for HIV-positive clients, since these clients have a heightened sense of the value of time.[85]

Past Trauma and HIV

The psychotherapeutic task of working with an HIV-positive person can be complicated by a history of trauma. HIV disease can be an event and a signifier, constituting both a loss, in and of itself, and a representation of previous losses. As such, it can reawaken painful and unintegrated affective states related to previous injuries. For example, for a woman with a history of sexual assault, HIV seroconversion became a window into feelings of helplessness, guilt about not fighting back, and of her own "badness." Conversely, newer traumas can stir up unresolved HIV-related issues. For a gay man who had been deeply dissatisfied with his long-term relationship, the end of this relationship generated profound anxiety, depression, and guilt. After considerable work in therapy, unresolved issues surfaced about his fear that he had infected his partner years earlier. His feelings of guilt had kept him in a dysfunctional relationship and provoked strong emotional reactions when the relationship finally ended.

Therapists should remain vigilant about the ways in which HIV can represent other unresolved issues. Often, conflicts about status as an HIV-infected person is a code for unresolved issues about a person's status as a stigmatized minority (for example, gay, African American, or drug user). When the trauma is significant, for instance, in the case of post-traumatic stress disorder, the therapeutic uncovering and reworking of the emotional material must proceed in an orderly fashion. The first priority is establishing the therapeutic alliance; next, therapy seeks to help the client develop a repertoire of coping strategies; finally, therapy begins the process of the emotional reworking of the trauma.

Psychotherapeutic Modalities and Styles

Contemporary psychotherapy is extremely diverse, informed by many theoretical orientations and an even wider array of practices. This section considers the use of psychotherapy and support groups as interventions in the management of HIV-related depression. It examines three broad categories of the discipline: cognitive-behavioral, interpersonal, and psychoanalytic-psychodynamic approaches. Within these general divisions there are many more variations, particularly among psychoanalytic approaches, than this chapter can cover.

Cognitive-Behavioral Psychotherapy

Cognitive-behavioral therapy has been proven to be a highly effective tool in the management of major depression and has been widely applied to HIV-related depression and anxiety.[14,86,87] Cognitive-behavioral therapy implicates a client's negative cognitions about himself and the world in the production of depressive states. Cognitions are the ideas that make up thinking, including images, ideas, and verbal material: for example, the belief, common among depressed individuals, that they are worthless or failures. A person constructs these cognitive schemas – interpretations of the self – using both external and internal information; in the context of depression, these schemas are negative and harsh and marked by expectations of failure and despair.

Cognitive therapies define depression in terms of a classical "cognitive triad" of schemas. The depressed person views himself as defective, worthless, and inadequate; perceives the world as negative and barren; and imagines the future as hopeless, marked always by failure and difficulty. Cognitive-behavioral theory posits that since the depressive schemas are basically learned, they can be unlearned, and since they are the engines for sustaining depression, changing them will improve mood.

Cognitive-behavioral therapy proceeds in a fairly systematized fashion. The therapist helps the client identify negative cognitions and test their validity. Does the client realize, for example, that he or she always expects rejection in the world? Is it true that the world is uniformly a harsh and unaccommodating place, or have there, in fact, been moments in the client's experience that contradict this distorted view? In many ways, the work of painstakingly sorting through negative perceptions and cognitions is empirical, something like the scientific method. The therapist encourages the client to identify assumptions about him or herself, assimilate and weigh them as evidence, and like psychological hypotheses, decide whether these negative assumptions really stand up to rigorous investigation.

Simply identifying cognitive distortions, however, will not magically alter the depressive situation. The goal of the therapy is to construct alternative understandings about self and the world. The ultimate purpose is not so much to summarily displace depressive views with happy ones, but rather, to introduce a more flexible thinking that moves the client away from reactive, automatic, negative responses. For example, a client who has recently developed HIV-related symptoms and now complains of depression might experience some of the following negative cognitions: "There is nothing that I can do but suffer with my illness." "I will always be sick." "I am a bad person who deserves this." "Since I am a weak person there is nothing to be done." During the course of a cognitive therapy, these perceptions might evolve: "Sometimes I feel ill, but there are things that I can do to take care of myself and help myself feel better." "I don't always feel bad, but when I do, I erroneously believe it will last forever." "I can learn ways of confronting difficult moments."

This approach of identifying and testing cognitions proceeds at two levels. First, therapy ferrets out automatic thoughts. For example, in the context of HIV-related depressions, it is not unusual for clients to have the automatic thought that if they disclose their HIV status to those who are close to them, they will be rejected. To help a client test and contradict this cognition, therapy might explore in detail the reactions of people to whom the client has already disclosed serostatus or another personal secret. For instance, after telling a close friend about his or her seroconversion, the friend may have indeed expressed shock, fear, and anger, but in the wake of these initial emotions, offered the client a great deal of support. The client may now want to tell family members, but have the depressive expectation they will be uniformly rejecting. Therapy may help expose the ways in which the client is inappropriately generalizing, selecting only the negative aspects of his or her experience with the friend and discounting the positive results.

As therapy elaborates a constellation of automatic thoughts and tests them for validity, the patterns that undergird these cognitions begin to emerge. This is the second level of exploration, which focuses on the underlying assumptions of automatic thinking. These assumptions are often deeply embedded – the maladaptive guiding principles of the client's life. For example, the underlying assumption of the client who fears disclosing serostatus may be that he or she deserves to be punished with HIV because of previous "bad" behavior. The fundamental process for dealing with these assumptions is similar to responding to automatic thinking: the therapist assists the client in testing the assumptions by challenging their validity. Why is it so important to rigidly adhere to moral codes? Might illness not be the result of chance and epidemiology?

Cognitive therapists take an active role in working with clients and often incorporate behavioral techniques as part of the therapy. Agendas for the session are usually set by the therapist, who keeps the work on track. The therapist is fairly directive, while maintaining a warm, empathic stance. Often therapists assign homework in which clients keep detailed track of their thoughts and feelings in journals. They might have clients actively test assumptions in particular situations or actively try out new behaviors. For example, if the client felt incapable of making contact with a friend because of depressive isolation, the therapist might help the client plan for this by breaking down the task into more attainable steps: first, calling the friend on the phone, then meeting only briefly before setting up a longer outing. The therapist and client might then evaluate the client's performance on these tasks, taking stock of expectations, affective states, cognitions, and outcomes. Sometimes the therapist will use role playing, allowing a chance to explore affects and cognitions in the therapy sessions.

In work with HIV-positive individuals, cognitive-behavioral approaches have often been combined with relaxation techniques, such as guided imagery, meditation, or progressive muscle relaxation, to reduce anxiety associated with depression. One study reported statistically significant reductions in anxiety, anger, and depression in a group of symptomatic HIV-positive individuals after a seven-week program that combined cognitive-behavioral therapy with relaxation, education, and coping skills trainings.[88] Employing a ten-week cognitive-behavioral stress management group, another study found that cognitive-behavioral therapy significantly decreased levels of dysphoria, anxiety, and total distress in individuals with HIV.[89] Follow-up found that the group intervention on social support and cognitive coping strategies improved mood symptoms, specifically finding that acceptance of HIV infection, in particular, promoted positive mood.[90] Cognitive-behavioral therapy has also been used effectively in combination with antidepressant medications.[91]

Perhaps one of the reasons cognitive-behavioral strategies have been helpful in the context of HIV-related depression has been because they foster active coping. Avoidant coping styles might well be the result of faulty negative cognitions such as the belief that once infected, the individual is a passive victim for whom nothing can be done. A cognitive approach analyzes and cautiously dismantles this thinking, replacing it with constructive alternatives. This in turn allows a more engaged and realistic approach to managing HIV disease. Behavioral techniques might emphasize greater socialization and the development of supportive networks, which are also protective against symptomatic depression.

Cognitive-behavioral approaches might be particularly helpful to clients in depressive crises at the milestones of HIV progression. At these times, clients may have greater needs for the sense of mastery and control that cognitive approaches can impart. The principles employed in identifying and testing cognitive assumptions might also be applied to attitudes about both antidepressant and HIV-related medications, and perhaps – since an important part of adherence relates to cognitive perceptions about the effects of medications – as part of a systematic appraisal of adherence difficulties.

Interpersonal Therapy

Interpersonal therapy is a treatment for major depression that emphasizes the connection between mood and life events, focusing on current interpersonal relationships and symptoms as well as social function, rather than on childhood developmental and personality issues.[92] Interpersonal therapists take an active, supportive, non-neutral, and hopeful stance. Therapy usually lasts from twelve to sixteen sessions.[93] Because interpersonal therapy is the only psychotherapeutic modality that has been demonstrated in clinical trials to have a statistically significant advantage for the treatment of HIV-positive individuals with depression, it deserves particular attention.[94]

In the initial stages of the treatment the therapist conducts a thorough evaluation along the lines of the medical model. The therapist then explicitly gives the client the "sick" role, overtly identifying both depression and HIV as illnesses that require intervention, and providing the client with relief from a sense that he or she is somehow inherently defective. Making a formal diagnosis and assigning the sick role also makes the client responsible for working to get better.[92] An important part of these role assignments is that the therapist takes on the position as educator about both depression and HIV, and actively encourages the client to negotiate the role as an "HIV patient" who will seek medical care and struggle with the complexities involved in this task. This approach requires the therapist to stay abreast of new developments in both the depression and HIV fields.

Therapy concentrates on the defined problem areas identified in the evaluation. Each problem area is categorized into one of four groups, all regarding relationship difficulties (hence the name, interpersonal): grief, interpersonal role disputes, role transitions, and interpersonal deficits. To focus treatment, the therapist explicitly links a client's presenting complaint to one of these problem areas.

"Grief" encompasses difficulties with bereavement after the death of a loved one. Bereavement, or mourning, carries special significance for many HIV-positive clients, who have often experienced devastating losses in their social networks due to HIV. Unresolved issues about the death of a loved one can become intimately connected to fears about the client's own health and premature death. This is a case where the term "depression" is particularly confusing, since feelings of sadness, anger, and helplessness are common, even necessary, in the process of mourning. "Complicated bereavement" is the term used to designate a mourning process that has begun to erode the capacities of the client, resulting in functional impairment. Typically, the client is either unable to effectively mourn or, conversely, is unable to cease mourning; in either case, the result is clinically significant depressive symptoms. The interpersonal therapist facilitates the process of a completed mourning by assisting the client to re-experience and acknowledge both positive and negative elements and memories of the lost relationship. The therapist may also explore the client's anticipation of his or her own death.

A "role dispute" occurs when people in a relationship have expectations of each other that do not correspond. The interpersonal therapist first helps clarify the conflicts and correlates them to the development of the depressive episode. Once the conflicts have been delineated, the therapist assists the client to resolutely confront the other party in the dispute, to brainstorm possible solutions (including the possible dissolution of the relationship), and to strategize their implementation. An HIV diagnosis can dramatically alter established roles and lead to conflict. Most notably, significant difficulties can arise in sexual relationships if one of the partners becomes HIV-positive. In serodiscordant couples, in which one partner is HIV-negative and the other HIV-positive, there may be disputes about frequency and spontaneity of sexual play, or regarding the negotiation of safer sex. The onset of a debilitating opportunistic infection or even more minor HIV-related symptoms can also cause serious conflicts with employers or colleagues if the client needs extended time off from work to recuperate. Similarly, disputes may arise between a client and his or her medical provider about medication side effects, when to start or discontinue aggressive treatment, or the use of "as needed" medications such as pain relievers.

A "role transition" is loosely defined as any change in social role; typically any major life event will occasion such a change. HIV provides a major catalyst for profound alterations in social roles. The very diagnosis of HIV can irrevocably transform an individual's identity overnight from "healthy person" to "patient," and, of course, HIV disease progression can mark other significant milestones that result in role transitions. Social roles provide support for an individual's sense of him or herself. Any successful transition from one way of seeing oneself to another entails a process of mourning. Major change is disrupting, and it is common for a person to experience a nostalgic longing for the "old way" of being. The interpersonal therapist facilitates an examination of positive and negative aspects of both the old and the new roles. For example, if a client has been forced to go on permanent disability, therapy might focus not only on grieving the loss of employment income and status, but also on appreciating the new abundance of time and the resulting opportunity to explore previously neglected parts of oneself. Because HIV generates so many significant life events, HIV-related interpersonal therapy could probably always take role transition as its point of departure.

Finally, "interpersonal deficits" include long-standing problems the client has in initiating and sustaining meaningful interpersonal relationships, usually related to personality and character issues. These clients are likely to have DSM-defined personality disorders. Because HIV infection so universally results in life events that can be assimilated under either grief, role disputes, or role transitions, interpersonal therapy researchers recommend virtually eliminating this category for HIV-positive clients with depression.[92]

Studies have shown that interpersonal therapy is effective for HIV-related depression, both as a substitute for and an adjunct to antidepressant medications, and both as an acute and maintenance intervention.[95] In one study, John Markowitz and his colleagues compared four psychotherapeutic interventions – interpersonal therapy, cognitive-behavioral therapy, supportive therapy, and supportive therapy with imipramine – in a sixteen-week randomized clinical trial.[96] Study subjects, both male and female, had been seropositive for at least six months and had clinically significant levels of depression. Subjects receiving interpersonal therapy or supportive therapy with imipramine had significantly greater improvement on depressive measures than did subjects receiving the cognitive-behavioral therapy or supportive therapy alone. The researchers postulate that interpersonal therapy may be more relevant to HIV-positive clients than cognitive-behavioral therapy: the latter implicitly asks clients to change their negative cognitions about themselves and the world, but in the context of HIV disease, these negative cognitions may be true rather than distorted.[94]

By prioritizing the effects of life events on relationships, interpersonal therapy maintains a strong psychosocial perspective. Within this frame, the interpersonal therapist could easily blend in material from a wider cultural analysis. For example, interpersonal therapy might be particularly well suited to clients who are immigrants, because they necessarily experience dramatic role transitions as part of the immigration process.[97]

Psychodynamic Psychotherapy

Psychodynamic therapy is a broad therapeutic category, which uses theory and technique adapted from the many developments within psychoanalysis. It is the oldest of the therapies discussed here, with its roots in the psychology developed by Freud about a hundred years ago. In general, psychodynamic approaches focus on the unconscious motivations that drive maladaptive patterns of relating, feeling, and thinking. In this respect, psychodynamic therapies attempt to get at the root cause of depressive symptoms, the reasons why cognitive distortions or interpersonal difficulties are established in the first place. Psychodynamic therapy posits that these repeated patterns are the products of past relationships, traumas, and internal conflicts. In other words, there are deeply personal reasons for the establishment and continuation of depression.

Because unconscious motivations are, by definition, not obvious, psychodynamic approaches must find ways of investigating and examining psychic material that is not readily available to the client. One of the most powerful methods for doing this is to investigate the therapeutic relationship itself. The therapist invites the client to directly voice and discuss thoughts and feelings about the therapist. The psychodynamic therapist connects the client's expectations and reactions about the therapeutic situation to the client's personal history. The psychodynamic therapist also magnifies unconscious material by leaving sessions unstructured and fostering "free association." Unlike cognitive and interpersonal therapies, psychodynamic approaches tend not to restrict the focus of the therapeutic work: neither sessions nor the overall therapy is limited to a problem area, and therapists encourage clients to say whatever comes to mind. The therapeutic encounter becomes an open field, out of which the client and therapist begin to notice, name, and explore patterns and repetitions. These techniques tend to make psychodynamic approaches open-ended in terms of length, although there are time-limited psychodynamic treatments, which do restrict the focus of the work to a specific problem area.

Much of the literature written on psychodynamic therapy in the context of HIV has focused on questions of loss and identity.[98-102] In this respect, psychodynamic therapy shares themes with interpersonal psychotherapy, in which grief and role transitions are two of the focus problem areas. A major difference between the two modalities is that psychodynamic approaches tie current issues to the past, particularly to childhood developments. This results, for example, in the linking of the contemporary loss of a partner to early traumatic abandonments.

Open-ended psychodynamic therapies may be especially suited to clients presenting with clinical depression in the context of other emotional difficulties. Individuals who have suffered multiple or severe traumas – including childhood sexual and physical abuse or multiple losses of close friends and partners – require highly secure therapeutic environments in which to begin to heal. Shorter-term, problem-focused therapies may not afford the development of sufficient trust for the vulnerable work of re-experiencing painful emotions. This group of clients includes those who have experienced devastating losses due to HIV and clients with personality disorders, especially those for whom issues of abandonment are prominent. In general, it is probably safe to say that many clients with chronic or life-long emotional difficulties who also have HIV will probably require longer-term therapies to adequately deal with the emotional issues that haunt them.

Ronald: Integrating Interventions

The treatment of HIV-related depression may unfold in a variety of ways depending on the context and the content of a client's depression, a provider's therapeutic orientation, and the responsiveness of the depression to psychopharmacological treatment, among other factors. The hypothetical case of Ronald offers some insights into integrating interventions to achieve the best outcome.

A week after beginning HIV antiviral treatment, "Ronald," a 40-year-old, African American gay man, showed up tearful and agitated at the office of his primary care physician, "Emily Rosin, MD." He had been ruminating about the breakup with his boyfriend a month earlier, felt worthless, was unable to sleep (often awakening at 4:00 am), and had been having recurrent thoughts of jumping from the roof of his building. In addition, although Ronald did not complain of side effects from his HIV antiviral regimen, he said he could not continue them. "It's no use, it's no use," he kept repeating.

Dr. Rosin thoroughly inquired into Ronald's suicidal ideation. While he was clearly very distraught, she concluded that he had no specific intention to take his life: the suicidal thoughts scared Ronald. He had never actually seriously contemplated nor attempted suicide before, and he said he was able to use the emergency hotline numbers that Dr. Rosin provided should his suicidal impulse intensify. Ronald had no history of psychiatric illness, hospitalizations, or medication trials, and no history of substance use. Dr. Rosin suggested stopping the HIV medications and prescribed low-dose lorazepam (Ativan), an antianxiety agent. She then made an urgent referral to a colleague, psychiatrist "William Klein, MD."

When Ronald arrived in Dr. Klein's office two days later, his situation had improved only minimally. The lorazepam had helped a little with the severe insomnia and daytime anxiety, but Ronald remained distraught. He cried several times a day and spent his time at home alone, usually in bed. He had not been to work for two weeks due to his inability to concentrate or control his mood. The suicidal thoughts had gotten worse. Ronald spent part of each day thinking about the morbid details of a suicide: his ex-partner's discovery of his body after a sleeping pill overdose, his family's anguished surprise, and his imagined peaceful repose. These thoughts became a reverie, and when he "came to," he said he felt frightened and ashamed.

In Dr. Klein's office, Ronald also felt embarrassed: having always prided himself on his strength and resilience, Ronald now felt beaten and weak. He was also extremely anxious: he sweated heavily during the session and his heart raced. Ronald's story slowly unfolded. He was the youngest of four children of a working class family. He was the first member of his family to have attended college, and then later to obtain an advanced degree in business. He had come out as gay to a few friends during college, but had never told his family. Three years previously, after testing for the first time, Ronald had been diagnosed with HIV. He decided that he could not let the diagnosis affect him and tried to put it behind him and "get on with life." He made an appointment with a physician, but later cancelled it and sought no further care. A year later he met a man, Eric, and started a relationship that was to last two years. He told Eric, who was seronegative, about his HIV status early in their dating. Eric strongly encouraged Ronald to go to a doctor, but Ronald did not like to talk about his condition. The couple began having difficulty, in part due to their mixed serostatus. Ronald finally made an appointment to see Dr. Rosin as the relationship was ending. Shortly after breaking up with Eric, with his CD4+ cell count nearing 200, Ronald started an antiviral regimen. The depressive feelings that had been brewing for the prior two months now broke to the surface, and Ronald found himself in an emotional crisis.

Establishing a Relationship and Prescribing Medications

Dr. Klein diagnosed Ronald with major depressive disorder and started treatment with 20 milligrams of the SSRI antidepressant paroxetine (Paxil). He continued Ronald on the lorazepam, which helped control the insomnia and significant anxiety. Therapy sessions were scheduled for twice a week at first, mostly concentrating on Ronald's suicidal ideation and the management of his depressive feelings. While Dr. Klein did not follow an exclusively cognitive-behavioral approach, he did incorporate many of these techniques. Ronald critically examined his cognitions and learned to use relaxation methods. He and Dr. Klein developed an extensive plan for dealing with the suicidal thoughts and reviewed accessible emergency resources, including Dr. Klein himself. The psychiatrist was active in other ways. He spoke with Dr. Rosin early in the treatment, and the two concurred that despite Ronald's lowered CD4+ cell count, this was not the time for him to restart an HIV antiviral regimen (he had stopped in response to Dr. Rosin's suggestion). Ronald would need to be more psychologically prepared in order for the treatment to be successful. Dr. Klein also worked with social service staff to ensure Ronald was financially covered during his period of temporary disability from work. This intensive crisis management allowed Ronald to avoid hospitalization. It also established a therapeutic alliance based on trust: Dr. Klein, Ronald thought, was there to help.

Two weeks into the treatment, Dr. Klein increased Ronald's dose of the paroxetine to 40 milligrams. Ronald experienced exhaustion at the higher dose, and complained of increased sweating and jitteriness. A week later, he had experienced no dramatic improvement in the pervasive depressed mood and anxiety, although his suicidality seemed less acute. Ronald was increasingly worried about his absence from work, however, which seemed to him to be further proof of his ineptitude and worthlessness, and he obsessed about how he might recover his lost relationship with Eric.

In the fourth week, pressed by Ronald's urgency, Dr. Klein decided to switch antidepressants, although he usually waited a full four weeks to six weeks to determine whether a trial had been effective at the therapeutic dose. He discussed a variety of options with Ronald – including the use of other SSRIs, mirtazapine (Remeron), and buproprion (Wellbutrin) – in this way seeking Ronald's active participation in the decision-making process. Based on the side effect profiles, they finally decided on the SSRI citalopram (Celexa). Dr. Klein simultaneously slowly lowered the dose of paroxetine while increasing the dose of citalopram. A week later, Dr, Klein also added buspirone (Buspar), a non-benzodiazepine antianxiety agent, slowly tapering off the lorazepam.

During this month of crisis intervention and intense focus on medications, Dr. Klein actively encouraged hope and patience while empathically reflecting back Ronald's emotions. As Ronald's suicidality became less acute, therapy focused more on the recently lost relationship. In this phase of psychotherapy, Dr. Klein employed techniques from interpersonal therapy, focusing on grief and mourning. Ronald's loss of Eric had been particularly jarring because it was through his partner that he had confronted his denial about HIV. When the two parted, Ronald was suddenly left alone with the reality of his illness. With Dr. Klein's help, Ronald was able to fully mourn the lost relationship: he expressed a deep sense of anger and betrayal, and the fear that he would never find someone again. Dr. Klein became Ronald's most important confidant, and this, in and of itself, gave Ronald hope that he might make a meaningful connection with someone else.

Dr. Klein employed psychiatric medications as a part of the psychotherapeutic process. These medications provided a measure of emotional stability that enabled Ronald to confront some difficult feelings. Rather than just making the depressive feelings "go away," the citalopram allowed Ronald to experience the sadness and anger that inevitably surfaced when reviewing his breakup with Eric. The medications made tolerable what had been overwhelming. Although carefully monitoring Ronald's reactions to the medications, Dr. Klein kept the focus on the psychosocial issues and emphasized the therapeutic work.

Approaching Sociocultural Issues

Two months into the treatment, Ronald returned to work, at first part-time. His presenting symptoms of tearfulness, depressed mood, insomnia, worthlessness, suicidality, and severe anxiety were largely resolved. Ronald continued to feel sad, anxious, and angry at times, but these emotions did not interfere with his day-to-day functioning. Therapy continued with a focus on issues related to work and social support. With Dr. Klein's encouragement, Ronald deepened his relationship with friends, who were concerned and supportive. Ronald also eventually told two of his closest siblings both about his being gay and his being HIV-infected. These were emotionally taxing and painful conversations, but Ronald found in these siblings a renewable and sustaining source of support.

After accommodating himself to his work schedule, Ronald decided it was time to begin aggressive HIV antiviral treatment. While he was anxious about the medications, especially of the daily reminder of his serostatus, he used psychotherapy to overcome these fears. Around this time, Ronald began to attend a support group for HIV-positive gay men and developed stronger ties with members of his church.

An important aspect of Ronald's treatment involved questions of ethnicity. Ronald had often struggled with complex issues of racial discrimination. When he had gone to college, he had separated himself from the African American community. His most recent partners, including Eric, had been White, as were many of his friends. He often felt that he could be gay with White people, but not with Black people. He had felt guilty about succeeding financially, where his family had not, and guilty about his homosexuality. At times, HIV seemed a kind of punishment to Ronald for leaving his family behind. Dr. Klein was not African American, and as the treatment progressed he was not shy about putting this rather obvious fact on the table in the therapy. This difference became a powerful way of untangling and understanding the ways in which race, homosexuality, and HIV overlapped for Ronald.

Ronald's case illustrates a number of important issues. First, treatment always occurs in the context of a clinical relationship. Relationships with both Dr. Rosin and with Dr. Klein were instrumental in allowing Ronald a place of trust and safety in which to deal with highly sensitive issues. Second, the collaboration between Drs. Rosin and Klein enabled the formulation of a treatment plan that positioned Ronald as a whole person rather than as either a set of lab values or of untethered emotions. In the treatment with Dr. Klein, antidepressant and antianxiety medications were used judiciously as part of a comprehensive approach that married psychological and biological interventions, and that saw these interventions as complementary rather than contradictory. Finally the sociocultural elements of the case were developed both within psychotherapy, by investigating racial issues within the therapeutic dyad, and without, by fostering the deepening of social supports through Ronald's friends, family, support groups, and the church.

Conclusion

In the context of HIV disease, it is common for social service, primary care, and mental health providers to confront a wide range of depressive moods and symptoms in the clients they serve. It is both natural and healthy for individuals who are HIV-infected to express their distress about the many traumatic events that unfold over the course of an illness that affects an individual at every possible level of existence: as a biological force that disrupts the body's normal functioning; as a psychological trauma that causes discomfort or pain and radically changes self-concept; and as a cultural marker that disturbs social relationships with the burdens of fear, guilt, and stigma. Providers must make room for these natural feelings of distress and acknowledge them with empathy and compassion. But when HIV-related depressive feelings do not resolve through a natural process of accommodation, they rise to the level of symptoms of a clinical disorder and require intervention.

The accurate assessment of depressive symptoms is central, because diagnostic formulation determines treatment. However, depressive symptoms may be masked by HIV disease symptoms, and HIV-related conditions may mimic symptoms of clinical depression. This confusion most often occurs at the biological level, and depressive symptoms are often dismissed as the natural consequence of being ill. For example, mistaking HIV, rather than depression, for the cause of symptoms such as fatigue or appetite loss, has probably led to undertreatment of clinical depression in HIV-positive individuals. This is a particularly unfortunate occurrence in an age when antidepressant treatment is relatively inexpensive, effective, and safe.

Providers of HIV services should be sensitive to complaints of depression – or their disguised surrogates such as fatigue or self-medication via drug use – and be prepared to investigate them further. The DSM-IV diagnostic criteria for a major depressive episode form the backbone of this evaluation, and give front-line providers standards by which to judge the need for a more extensive psychiatric assessment. A careful exploration of symptoms should nonetheless extend beyond a simple checklist approach to include a full evaluation at all three levels of the biopsychosocial model. Providers should assess: biomedical manifestations of HIV, including opportunistic infections and medication side effects; psychosocial components, including an individual's coping style and the extent and resiliency of his or her social supports; and sociocultural factors, including the influence of stigma and marginalization, and the more traditional cultural questions of gender, sexuality, race, and ethnicity. If there is an indication of a clinical depression, formal psychiatric assessment may lead to a DSM diagnosis of major depression, dysthymia, bipolar disorder, an adjustment disorder, acute and post-traumatic stress disorder, or a personality disorder.

The cornerstone of treatment for clinical depression is medication management, psychotherapy, and support. Primary care providers and psychiatrists can make a determination as to the utility of antidepressant medication, prescribing it for any of the major depressive disorders found in the DSM. They may also recommend ancillary medications for anxiety, sleep disturbance, mood stabilization, or hormonal imbalances. But intervention should not end with medication management. A good general rule is that any client with sufficient symptomatology to take medication will probably also benefit from psychotherapy. Psychotherapy provides a relationship of trust in which the client can experience and work through difficult, sometimes overwhelming, emotions. Psychotherapy and medication management go hand in hand: medications stabilize the client sufficiently to allow the work of psychotherapy to proceed.

Finally, treatment should incorporate a sense of the sociocultural aspects of HIV. In both the medical and the mental health treatment relationships, providers should keep in mind the effects of stigma and marginalization. Every treatment plan for HIV-related depression should include an attempt to broaden or deepen social connections, whether through existing networks of friends and family or through newly established ones such as support groups.

HIV and depression have been intimately related since the beginning of the epidemic. But, where there was once panic, ostracism, and helplessness, there is now knowledge, support, and hope. HIV remains a potentially devastating and often terrifying disease, but increasingly, it can be managed and controlled. At the same time as HIV treatment has improved, so has treatment for depression. It is these two messages that should inform the thinking of providers: clinical levels of depression should not be seen as "normal" or expected outcomes of having HIV disease, and clinical depression is eminently treatable.

References

1. Catalan J. Psychosocial and neuropsychiatric aspects of HIV infection: Review of their extent and implications for psychiatry. *Journal of Psychosomatic Research.* 1988; 32(3): 237-248.

2. Marzuk PM, Tierney H, Tardiff K, et al. Increased risk of suicide in persons with AIDS. *Journal of the American Medical Association.* 1988; 259(9): 1333-1337.

3. Kizer KW, Green M, Perkins CI, et al. AIDS and suicide in California. *Journal of the American Medical Association.* 1988; 260(13): 1881.

4. Lyketsos CG, Treisman GJ. Depressive syndromes and causal associations. *Psychosomatics.* 1996; 37(5): 407-412.

5. Coté TR, Biggar RJ, Dannenberg AL. Risk of suicide among persons with AIDS: A national assessment. *Journal of the American Medical Association.* 1992; 268(15): 2066-2068.

6. Rabkin JG, Ferrando SJ, Jacobsberg LB, et al. Prevalence of Axis I disorders in an AIDS cohort: A cross-sectional, controlled study. *Comprehensive Psychiatry.* 1997; 38(3): 146-154.

7. Rabkin JG, Remien RH. Depressive disorder and HIV disease: An uncommon association. *FOCUS: A Guide to AIDS Research and Counseling.* 1995; 10(9): 1-4.

8. Styron W. *Darkness Visible: A Memoir of Madness.* New York: Vintage Books, 1990.

9. Page-Shafer K, Delorenze GN, Satariano WA, et al. Comorbidity and survival in HIV-infected men in the San Francisco Men's Health Survey. *Annals of Epidemiology.* 1996; 6(5): 420-430.

10. Singh N, Squier C, Sivek C, et al. Determinants of compliance with antiretroviral therapy in patients with human immunodeficiency virus: Prospective assessment with implications for enhancing compliance. *AIDS Care.* 1996; 8(3): 261-269.

11. DiMatteo MR, Lepper HS, Croghan TW. Depression is a risk factor for noncompliance with medical treatment: Meta-analysis of the effects of anxiety and depression on patient adherence. *Archives of Internal Medicine.* 2000; 160(14): 2101-2107.

12. Katz MH, Douglas JM Jr, Bolan GA, et al. Depression and use of mental health services among HIV-infected men. *AIDS Care.* 1996; 8(4): 433-442.

13. American Psychiatric Association. *Diagnostic and Statistical Manual of Mental Disorders.* 4th edition. Washington, D.C.: American Psychiatric Association, 1994.

14. Kaplan HI, Sadock BJ, Grebb JA, eds. *Kaplan and Sadock's Synopsis of Psychiatry.* 7th edition. Baltimore: Lippincott, Williams and Wilkins, 1994.

15. Kalichman SC, Sikkema KJ, Somlai A. Assessing persons with human immunodeficiency virus (HIV) infection using the Beck Depression Inventory: Disease processes and other potential confounds. *Journal of Personality Assessment.* 1995; 64(1): 86-100.

16. Ostrow DG, Monjan A, Joseph J, et al. HIV-related symptoms and psychological functioning in a cohort of homosexual men. *American Journal of Psychiatry.* 1989; 146(6): 737-742.

17. Burrack JH, Barrett DC, Stall R, et al. Depressive symptoms and CD4 lymphocyte decline among HIV-infected men. *Journal of the American Medical Association.* 1993; 270(21): 2568-2578.

18. Lyketsos CG, Hoover DR, Guccione M, et al. Depressive symptoms as predictors of medical outcomes in HIV infection. *Journal of the American Medical Association*. 1993; 270(21): 2563-2567.

19. Drebing CE, Van Gorp WG, Hinkin C, et al. Confounding factors in the measurement of depression in HIV. *Journal of Personality Assessment*. 1994; 62(1): 68-83.

20. Lyketsos CG, Treisman GJ. Depressive syndromes and causal associations. *Psychosomatics*. 1996; 37(5): 407-412.

21. Maj M. Depressive syndromes and symptoms in subjects with human immunodeficiency virus (HIV) infection. *British Journal of Psychiatry*. 1996; 168(30): 117-122.

22. Dew MA, Becker JT, Sanchez J, et al. Prevalence and predictors of depressive, anxiety, and substance use disorders in HIV-infected and uninfected men: A longitudinal evaluation. *Psychological Medicine*. 1997; 27(2): 395-409.

23. Ostrow DG, Monjan A, Joseph J, et al. HIV-related symptoms and psychological functioning in a cohort of homosexual men. *American Journal of Psychiatry*. 1989; 146(6): 737-742.

24. Lyketsos CG, Hoover DR, Guccione M, et al. Depressive symptoms as predictors of medical outcomes in HIV infection. *Journal of the American Medical Association*. 1993; 270(21): 2563-2567.

25. Kathol RG, Noyes R, Williams J, et al. Diagnosing depression in patients with medical illness. *Psychosomatics*. 1990; 31(4): 434-440.

26. Breitbart W, McDonald MV, Rosenfeld B, et al. Fatigue in ambulatory AIDS patients. *Journal of Pain and Symptom Management*. 1998; 15(3): 159-167.

27. Ferrando S, Evans S, Goggin K, et al. Fatigue in HIV illness: Relationship to depression, physical limitations, and disability. *Psychosomatic Medicine*. 1998; 60(6): 759-764.

28. Rubinstein ML, Selwyn PA. High prevalence of insomnia in an outpatient population with HIV infection. *Journal of Acquired Immune Deficiency Syndromes and Human Retrovirology*. 1998; 19(3): 260-265.

29. White JL, Merrill MM, Darko DF. Sleep disturbance in early HIV infection. *FOCUS: A Guide to AIDS Research and Counseling*. 1995; 10(11): 5-6.

30. Groopman JE. Fatigue in cancer and HIV/AIDS. *Oncology*. 1998; 12(3): 335-344.

31. Goggin KJ, Zisook S, Heaton RK, et al. Neuropsychological performance of HIV-1 infected men with major depression. *Journal of the International Neuropsychological Society*. 1997; 3(5): 457-464.

32. Goldblum PB, Erickson S. *Working with AIDS Bereavement: A Comprehensive Approach for Mental Health Providers*. San Francisco: UCSF AIDS Health Project, 1999.

33. Hays RB, Turner H, Coates TJ. Social support, AIDS-related symptoms, and depression among gay men. *Journal of Consulting and Clinical Psychology*. 1992; 60(3): 463-469.

34. Lackner JB, Joseph JG, Ostrow DG, et al. The effects of social support on Hopkins Symptom Checklist-assessed depression and distress in a cohort of human immunodeficiency virus-positive and -negative gay men. *Journal of Nervous and Mental Diseases*. 1993; 181(10): 632-638.

35. Belkin GS, Fleishman JA, Stein MD, et al. Physical symptoms and depressive symptoms among individuals with HIV infection. *Psychosomatics*. 1992; 33(4): 416-425.

36. Kelly JA, Murphy DA, Bahr GR, et al. Factors associated with severity of depression and high-risk sexual behavior among persons diagnosed with human immunodeficiency virus (HIV) infection. *Health Psychology*. 1993; 12(3): 215-219.

37. Cohen S, McKay G. Social support, stress, and the buffering hypothesis: A theoretical analysis. In Baum A, Singer JE, Taylor SE, eds. *Handbook of Psychology and Health, Volume 4*. Hilldale, NJ: Lawrence Erlbaum Associates, 1984.

38. Atkinson JH, Grant I, Kennedy CJ, et al. Prevalence of psychiatric disorders among men infected with human immunodeficiency virus: A controlled study. *Archives of General Psychiatry*. 1988; 45(9): 859-864.

39. Perry S, Jacobsberg LB, Fishman B, et al. Psychiatric diagnosis before serological testing for the human immunodeficiency virus. *American Journal of Psychiatry* 1990; 147(1): 89-93.

40. Rosenberger PH, Bornstein RA, Nasrallah HA, et al. Psychopathology in human immunodeficiency virus infection: Lifetime and current assessment. *Comprehensive Psychiatry*. 1993; 34(3): 150-158.

41. Williams JW, Rabkin JG, Remien RH, et al. Multidisciplinary baseline assessment of homosexual men with and without HIV infection. II. Standardized clinical assessment of current and lifetime psychopathology. *Archives of General Psychiatry*. 1991; 48(2): 124-130.

42. Maj M. Depressive syndromes and symptoms in subjects with human immunodeficiency virus (HIV) infection. *British Journal of Psychiatry*. 1996; 168(30): 117-122.

43. Cohen M, Furumoto-Dawson A, Koshy R, et al. Identifying and treating mental health problems in women with HIV: Lessons from a woman-centered program. Presentation from the Third National Conference on Women and HIV, Pasadena, California, May 1997.

44. Kaplan MS, Marks G, Mertens SB. Distress and coping among women with HIV infection: Preliminary findings from a multiethnic sample. *American Journal of Orthopsychiatry*. 1997; 67(1): 80-91.

45. Dew MA, Blechman IJ, Sanchez J, et al. Prevalence of psychiatric disorders and factors affecting mental health services utilization in a primary care population of HIV+ women. Presentation from the Third National Conference on Women and HIV, Pasadena, California, May 1997.

46. Pergami A, Gala C, Burgess A, et al. The psychological impact of HIV infection in women. *Journal of Psychosomatic Research*. 1993; 37(7): 687-696.

47. Siegle K, Karus D, Ravels VH, et al. Psychological adjustment of women with HIV/AIDS: Racial and ethnic comparisons. *Journal of Community Psychology*. 1998; 26(5): 439-455.

48. Ferrando S, Rabkin JG, Heller D, et al. Treatment of depression in HIV positive women. Presentation from the XII World AIDS Conference, Geneva, Switzerland, June 1998.

49. Moneyham L, Seals B, Demi A, et al. Perceptions of stigma in women infected with HIV. *AIDS Patient Care and STDs*. 1996; 10(3): 162-167.

50. Smeltzer SC, Whipple B. Women and HIV infection. *Image*. 1991; 23: 249-255.

51. Richardson J, Barkan S, Cohen M, et al. Experience and covariates among a cohort of HIV-infected women. Presentation from the XI International Conference on AIDS, Vancouver, Canada, July 1996.

52. Nelson WL, Ferrando SJ, Stanislawski DM, et al. Childhood trauma, substance abuse, and distress in HIV-infected women. Presentation from the XI International Conference on AIDS, Vancouver, Canada, July 1996.

53. Weiner LS. Women and human immunodeficiency virus. *Social Work*. 1991; 36(1): 375-378.

54. Martinez Y. Sexual silence: To battle AIDS, Hispanics must overcome cultural barriers. *Hispanic.* 1997; 10(1-2): 100-104.

55. Rabkin JG, Lin H, Lipsitz J, et al. Psychopathology in male and female HIV positive and negative injecting drug users: Longitudinal course over 3 years. *AIDS.* 1997; 11(4): 507-515.

56. Lipsitz J, Williams JB, Rabkin JG, et al. Psychopathology in male and female intravenous drug users with and without HIV infection. *American Journal of Psychiatry.* 1994; 151(11): 1662-1668.

57. Altice F, Khooshnood K, Blankenship KM, et al. Health status and co-morbidity of HIV and HIV-out-of-treatment injection drug users. Presentation from the XII World AIDS Conference, Geneva, Switzerland, June 1998.

58. Davis RF, Metzger DS, Meyers K, et al. Long-term changes in psychological symptomatology associated with HIV serostatus among male injecting drug users. *AIDS.* 1995; 9(1): 73-79.

59. Hawkins WE, Latkin C, Hawkins MJ, et al. Depressive symptoms and HIV-risk behavior in inner-city users of injection drugs. *Psychological Reports.* 1998; 82(1): 137-138.

60. Latkin CA, Mandell W. Depression as an antecedent of frequency of intravenous drug use in an urban, non-treatment sample. *International Journal of Addictions.* 1993; 28(14): 1601-1612.

61. Nelson WL, Ferrando SJ, Stanislawski DM, et al. Childhood trauma, substance abuse, and distress in HIV-infected women. Presentation from the XI International Conference on AIDS, Vancouver, Canada, July 1996.

62. Wang MQ, Collins CB, DiClemente RJ, et al. Depressive symptoms as correlates of polydrug use for blacks in a high-risk community. *Southern Medical Journal.* 1997; 90(11): 1123-1128.

63. Booth RE, Koester SK, Pinto F. Gender differences in sex-risk behaviors, economic livelihood, and self-concept among drug injectors and crack smokers. *American Journal on Addictions.* 1995; 4(4): 313-322.

64. Nemoto T, Foster K, Brown LS. Effect of psychological factors on risk behavior of human immunodeficiency virus (HIV) infection among intravenous drug users (IVDUs). *International Journal of Addictions.* 1991; 26(4): 441-456.

65. Diaz RM. *Latino Gay Men and HIV: Culture, Sexuality, and Risk Behavior.* New York: Routledge, 1998.

66. Spalding AD. Racial minorities and other high-risk groups with HIV and AIDS at increased risk for psychological adjustment problems in association with health locus of control orientation. *Social Work in Health Care.* 1995; 21(3): 81-114.

67. Peterson JL, Folkman S, Bakeman R. Stress, coping, HIV status, psychosocial resources, and depressive mood in African American gay, bisexual, and heterosexual men. *American Journal of Community Psychology.* 1996; 24(4): 461-487.

68. Cochran SD, Mays VM. Depressive distress among homosexually active African American men and women. *American Journal of Psychiatry.* 1994; 151(4): 524-529.

69. Public Media Center. *AIDS Stigma and Discrimination: The Attitudes of National Experts and Influentials.* San Francisco: Communication Technologies, n.d.

70. Treichler PA. AIDS, homophobia, and biomedical discourse: An epidemic of signification. In Crimp D, ed. *AIDS: Cultural Analysis, Cultural Activism.* Cambridge, Mass.: MIT Press, 1988.

71. Singh N, Squier C, Sivek C, et al. Determinates of compliance with antiretroviral therapy in patients with human immunodeficiency virus: Prospective assessment with implications for enhancing compliance. *AIDS Care.* 1996; 8(3): 261-269.

72. Cabaj RP. Substance abuse in gay men, lesbians, and bisexuals. In Cabaj RP, Stein TS, eds. *Textbook of Homosexuality and Mental Health.* Washington, D.C.: American Psychiatric Press, Inc., 1996.

73. *HIV and the Central Nervous System: Part One and HIV and the Central Nervous System: Part Two.* CNS Spectrums, 2000; 5(4-5).

74. Kathol RG, Noyes R, Williams J, et al. Diagnosing depression in patients with medical illness. *Psychosomatics,* 1990; 31(4): 434-440.

75. Lazarus A. AIDS mania: Review and case report. *Annals of Clinical Psychiatry.* 1992; 4(4): 301-304.

76. Rabkin JG, Remien R. Katoff L, et al. Resilience in adversity among long-term survivors of AIDS. *Hospital and Community Psychiatry.* 1993; 44(2): 162-167.

77. Rabkin JG, Wagner GJ, Rabkin R. Fluoxetine treatment for depression in patients with HIV and AIDS: A randomized, placebo-controlled trial. *American Journal of Psychiatry.* 1999; 156(1): 101-107.

78. Elliott AJ, Uldall KK, Bergam K, et al. Randomized, placebo-controlled trial of paroxetine versus imipramine in depressed HIV-positive outpatients. *American Journal of Psychiatry.* 1998; 155(3): 367-372.

79. Pies RW. *Handbook of Essential Psychopharmacology.* Washington, D.C.: American Psychiatric Press, Inc., 1998.

80. Wagner GJ, Maguen S, Rabkin JG. Ethnic differences in response to fluoxetine in a controlled trial with depressed HIV-positive patients. *Psychiatric Services.* 1998; 49(2): 239-240.

81. Fernandez F, Levy JK, Galizzi H. Response of HIV-related depression to psychostimulants: Case reports. *Hospital and Community Psychiatry.* 1988; 39(6): 628-631.

82. Esch J, Breitbart B, Rosenfeld B, et al. Psychostimulants for fatigue in the HIV positive patient: Placebo controlled trial of methylphenidate and pemoline. Presentation from the XII World AIDS Conference, Geneva, Switzerland, June 1998.

83. Rabkin JG, Wagner GJ, Rabkin R. Testosterone therapy for human immunodeficiency virus-positive men with and without hypogonadism. *Journal of Clinical Psychopharmacology.* 1999; 19(1): 19-27.

84. Ziefert P, Leary M, Boccalari A. *AIDS and the Impact of Cognitive Impairment: A Treatment Guide for Mental Health Professionals.* San Francisco: UCSF AIDS Health Project, 1995.

85. Devine J. The role of psychotherapy in coping with HIV disease. In Dilley JW, Marks R, eds. *The UCSF AIDS Health Project Guide to Counseling: Perspectives on Psychotherapy, Prevention and Therapeutic Practice.* San Francisco: Jossey-Bass Publishers, 1998.

86. Beck AT, Rush AJ, Shaw BF, et al. *Cognitive Therapy of Depression.* New York: Guilford Press, 1979.

87. Shaw B, Segal ZV. Introduction to cognitive theory and therapy. In Frances AJ, Hales RE, eds. *American Psychiatric Press Review of Psychiatry,* Volume 7. Washington, D.C.: American Psychiatric Press, Inc., 1988.

88. Inouye J, Flannelly L, Flannelly KJ. Reducing emotional distress in individuals who are HIV-positive. Presentation from the XII World AIDS Conference, Geneva, Switzerland, June 1998.

89. Lutgendorf SK, Antonni MH, Ironson G, et al. Cognitive-behavioral stress management decreases dysphoric mood and herpes simplex virus-type 2 antibody titers in symptomatic HIV-seropositive gay men. *Journal of Consulting and Clinical Psychology.* 1997; 65(1): 31-43.

90. Lutgendorf SK, Antonni MH, Ironson G, et al. Changes in cognitive coping skills and social support during cognitive behavioral stress management intervention and distress outcomes in symptomatic immunodeficiency virus (HIV)-seropositive gay men. *Psychosomatic Medicine.* 1998; 60(2): 204-214.

91. Lee MR, Cohen L, Hadley SW, et al. Cognitive-behavioral group therapy with medication for depressed gay men with AIDS or symptomatic HIV infection. *Psychiatric Services.* 1999; 50(7): 948-952.

92. Klerman GL, Weissman MM, Rounsaville BJ, et al. *Interpersonal Psychotherapy of Depression.* New York: Basic Books, 1984.

93. Swartz HA, Markowitz JC. Interpersonal psychotherapy for the treatment of depression in HIV-positive men and women. In Markowitz JC, ed. *Interpersonal Psychotherapy.* Washington, D.C.: American Psychiatric Press, Inc., 1998.

94. Markowitz JC, Klerman GL, Clougherty KF, et al. Individual psychotherapies for depressed HIV-positive patients. *American Journal of Psychiatry.* 1995; 152(10): 1504-1509.

95. Weissman MN. Interpersonal psychotherapy: Current status. *Keio Journal of Medicine.* 1997; 46(3): 105-110.

96. Markowitz JC, Kocsis JH, Fishman B, et al. Treatment of depressive symptoms in human immunodeficiency virus-positive patients. *Archives of General Psychiatry.* 1998; 55(5): 452-457.

97. Armas R, personal communication, September 2000.

98. Weiss JJ. Psychotherapy with HIV-positive gay men: A psychodynamic perspective. *American Journal of Psychotherapy.* 1997; 51(1): 31-44.

99. Nord D. Threats to identity in survivors of multiple AIDS-related losses. *American Journal of Psychotherapy.* 1997; 51(3): 387-402.

100. Blechner MJ, ed. *Hope and Mortality: Psychodynamic Approaches to AIDS and HIV.* Hillsdale, N.J.: The Analytic Press, 1997.

101. Hildebrand, HP. A patient dying with AIDS. *International Review of Psycho-Analysis.* 1992, 19(4): 457-469.

102. Cadwell SA, Burnham RA, Forstein M, eds. *Therapists on the Front Line: Psychotherapy with Gay Men in the Age of AIDS.* Washington, D.C.: American Psychiatric Press, Inc., 1994.

Resources

Included here are general mental health resources and HIV-related mental health resources from six HIV epicenters in the United States: Chicago, Houston, Los Angeles, Miami, New York, and San Francisco.

General Resources

Alcoholics Anonymous (AA), General Services Office, Box 459, Grand Central Station, New York, New York 10163, 212-870-3400, www.alcoholics-anonymous.org. *Provides literature and audiovisual materials on alcoholism and AA.*

American Psychiatric Association, 1400 K Street, NW, Washington, DC 20005, 888-357-7924, Fax 202-682-6850, www.psych.org. *Provides referrals and publications.*

American Psychological Association, 750 First Street, NE, Washington, DC 20002-4242, 800-374-2721, 202-336-5500, Referrals 800-964-2000, www.apa.org. *Provides referrals and publications.*

Narcotics Anonymous (NA) World Service Organization, P.O. Box 9999, Van Nuys, California 92409, 818-773-9999, www.na.org. *Produces newsletters and publications.*

National Alliance for the Mentally Ill (NAMI), Colonial Place Three, 2107 Wilson Boulevard, Suite 300, Arlington, Virginia 22201-3042, 703-524-7600, HelpLine 800-950-6264, Fax 703-524-9094, www.nami.org. *Provides information, support, and advocacy to people with severe mental illness and their friends and families.*

National Institute of Mental Health (NIMH), Public Inquiries, 6001 Executive Boulevard, Room 8184, MSC 9663, Bethesda, MD 20892-9663, 301-443-4513, Fax 301-443-4279, www.nimh.nih.gov/publicat/aidsmenu.cfm. *Provides research and literature on HIV and mental health.*

National Mental Health Association, 1021 Prince Street, Alexandria, Virginia, 22314, 800-228-1114, www.nmha.org. *Provides a clearinghouse of mental health facilities regionally.*

Chicago Area

Howard Brown Health Center, 4025 North Sheridan Road, Chicago, Illinois 60613, 773-388-1600, www.howardbrown.org. *Provides case management for HIV-positive clients, individual and group therapy, and support groups.*

Pride Institute, 4840 North Marine Drive, Chicago, Illinois 60640, 773-907-4594, www.pride-institute.com. *Provides mental health services to people with HIV.*

Test Positive Aware Network (TPAN), 1258 West Belmont, Chicago, Illinois 60657, 773-404-8726, Fax 773-404-1040, www.tpan.com. *Provides support groups for people with HIV.*

Houston Area

Montrose Counseling Center, 701 Richmond Avenue, Houston, Texas 77006, 713-520-0037, Fax 713-526-4367, www.neosoft.com/~mcc. *Provides individual, couples, family, and group therapy for people with HIV.*

Chicano Family Center, 7524 Avenue E, Houston, Texas 77012, 713-923-2316, Fax 713-923-4243. *Provides mental health services in Spanish and English to people with HIV.*

Los Angeles Area

AIDS Project Los Angeles (APLA), 1313 North Vine Street, Los Angeles, California 90028, 323-993-1600, Fax 323-993-1598, www.apla.org. *Provides counseling for clients with HIV-related mental health problems.*

AIDS Service Center, 1030 South Arroyo Parkway, Pasadena, California 91105, 626-441-8495, www.aidsservicecenter.org. *Provides mental health services for people with HIV.*

Tarzana Treatment Center, Reseda Facility, 7101 Baird Avenue, Reseda, California 91335, 818-342-5897, www.tarzanatc.org. *Provides counseling services for individuals and families.*

Miami Area

Care Resource, 1320 South Dixie Highway, Suite 485, Coral Gables, Florida 33146, 305-667-9296, Fax 305-667-8686, www.careresource.net. *Offers counseling services for HIV-positive individuals and their families in English and Spanish.*

Center for Positive Connections, 12570 NE 7th Avenue, #104, North Miami, Florida 33161, 305-891-2066, 888-POS-CONN, Fax 305-891-5053, www.positiveconnections.org. *Provides emotional and social support, targeting heterosexuals, newly diagnosed, affected family and friends.*

Family Counseling Services of Greater Miami, 10651 North Kendall Drive, Suite 100, Miami, Florida 33176, 305-271-9800, Fax 305-270-3330, www.familycounseling. org/contact.htm. *Provides family, couples, and individual counseling.*

New York Area

Asian and Pacific Islander Coalition on HIV/AIDS (APICHA), 275 Seventh Avenue, Suite 1204, New York, New York 10001, 212-620-7287, Fax 212-620-7323, www.apicha2.org/index.htm. *Offers support groups.*

Gay Men's Health Crisis (GMHC), 119 West 24th Street, New York, New York 10011, 212-807-6664, Hotline 212-807-6655, www.gmhc.org. *Offers HIV-related peer counseling, support groups, and individual therapy.*

Identity House, 39 West 14th Street, Suite 205, New York, New York 10011, 212-243-8181, www.erols.com/identityhouse. *Provides individual and couples counseling for people with HIV.*

Institute for Human Identity, 160 West 24th Street, New York, New York 10011, 212-243-2830, Fax 212-243-3175. *Provides mental health services for people with HIV.*

San Francisco Area

Center for Special Problems, 1700 Jackson Street, San Francisco, California 94109, 415-292-1500, Fax 415-292-2030. *Provides individual and group therapy for people with HIV.*

Instituto Familiar De La Raza, 2919 Mission Street, San Francisco, California 94110, 415-647-4141, Fax 415-647-3662. *Provides mental health services in Spanish and English for people with HIV.*

New Leaf, 1853 Market Street, San Francisco, California 94103, 415-626-7000, 415-626-5916, www.newleafservices.org. *Provides HIV-related outpatient therapy.*

UCSF AIDS Health Project, Box 0884, San Francisco, California 94143-0884, 415-476-3902, www.ucsf-ahp.org. *Provides mental health services for HIV-positive and HIV-negative clients. Offers consultation and training to mental health providers.*

Index